EMERGENCY PSYCHIATRY

DATE DUE

AUG 3 1 2005

NOTICE

EMERGENCY PSYCHIATRY

Randy Hillard, MD

Professor and Chairman, Department of Psychiatry
University of Cincinnati College of Medicine
Cincinnati, Ohio

Brook Zitek, DO
Assistant Professor
Department of Psychiatry
Temple University School of Medicine
Philadelphia, Pennsylvania

McGraw-Hill
Medical Publishing Division

New York   Chicago   San Francisco   Lisbon   London   Madrid   Mexico City
Milan   New Delhi   San Juan   Seoul   Singapore   Sydney   Toronto

Emergency Psychiatry

1 2 3 4 5 6 7 8 9 0   DOC/DOC   0 9 8 7 6 5 4 3

ISBN 0-07-141505-X

This book was set in Times Roman by Westchester Book Services.
The editors were Marc Strauss and Kathleen McCullough.
The production supervisor was Richard Ruzycka.
Project management was provided by Westchester Book Services.
The index was prepared by Sandi Schroeder.
RR Donnelley was printer and binder.

This book was printed on acid-free paper.

Library of Congress Cataloging-in-Publication Data

Emergency psychiatry / edited by Randy Hillard, Brook Zitek.—1st ed.
    p. ; cm.
   Includes bibliographical references and index.
   ISBN 0-07-141505-X
   1. Psychiatric emergencies.   2. Crisis intervention (Mental health services)   I. Hillard, Randy.   II. Zitek, Brook.
   [DNLM: 1. Emergency Services, Psychiatric—methods.   2. Diagnosis, Differential.
3. Mental Disorders—diagnosis.   4. Mental Disorders—therapy.   WM 401 E5311 2004]
RC480.6.E4432 2004
616.89'025—dc22   2003059320

CONTENTS

3. BIOLOGICAL TREATMENT PRINCIPLES   23

4. PSYCHOSOCIAL PRINCIPLES   41

5. LEGAL PRINCIPLES   49

6. PSYCHIATRIC ETHICS

Part II Clinical Challenges in Emergency Psychiatry

7. THE POTENTIALLY SUICIDAL PATIENT

8. THE POTENTIALLY VIOLENT PATIENT

9. MOOD/ANXIETY DISORDERS 91

10. SUBSTANCE USE DISORDERS 127

11. SCHIZOPHRENIA AND PSYCHOTIC DISORDERS 171

12. PERSONALITY DISORDERS 191

INDEX 227

PREFACE

Emergency psychiatry is a subspecialty of psychiatry that has evolved over the last few decades. In 1960, there were approximately 650,000 psychiatric inpatient beds in public facilities. By 2000, there were just 57,000 (*Psychiatric News* 2002). This decline in available hospital beds has created an upswing in the growth of psychiatric emergency services and mobile crisis teams, and in the number of psychiatric patients seen in community mental health and other less restrictive settings.

As inpatient psychiatry beds have been reduced throughout the United States, psychiatric emergency services have grown. With the growth of these services, the subspecialty of emergency psychiatry and the skill set required of such emergency clinicians has become more clearly defined. Many urban, university-based Psychiatric Emergency Service (PES) settings have become academic services filled with trainees of many disciplines including medicine, nursing, psychology, and social work. The PES is truly multispecialty dependent in order to run efficiently.

Emergency psychiatry is not only the realm of the PES setting, however. All mental health clinicians have been or will be faced with situations involving patients in crisis. The authors offer this clinical guide with the hope that it will provide help in dealing with such clinical situations.

Part I provides an introduction to the basic principles of emergency psychiatry. The authors include a chapter on the emergency medicine approach to psychiatric illness, a perspective offered by an emergency medicine physician.

Part II addresses the unique features of various psychiatric disorders and situations in the acute or emergency psychiatry phase. Much of the *Diagnostic and Statistical Manual of Mental Disorders*, 4th edition, Text Revision (DSM-IV-TR) is included in this guide, reorganized into what the authors hope to be a more user friendly and easily accessible table format. We do so in acknowledgement that this (the DSM) is our dictionary, our common language, and we want to keep diagnostic information consistent with the DSM.

Chapters on "The Potentially Suicidal Patient" and "The Potentially Violent Patient" are offered to address these particularly trying clinical challenges with attention to patient safety issues. "Mood/Anxiety Disorders," "Substance Use Disorders," "Schizophrenia and Psychotic Disorders," and "Personality Disorders" are each covered in separate chapters.

The authors gratefully acknowledge colleagues who offered suggestions and comments. Dr. William Dubin, Dr. David Baron, and Dr. Ralph Spiga in particular provided useful guidance regarding the writing process. Dr. Henry

Weisman and the respective staffs of the University of Cincinnati PES and the Temple Crisis Response Center provided collegial and supportive work environments. Marc Strauss, our editor at McGraw-Hill, was consistently available and skillfully guided the process.

We wish to thank our respective families for their support in this endeavor. Dr. Zitek is particularly grateful to her partner, Joan Lau, for unfailing patience, humor, and support in this process. Dr. Hillard thanks his wife, Aingeal Grehan, for her temperance and support.

The authors believe that the PES will continue to develop as an important training and research site, and specialty training/fellowship programs will continue to expand in kind. The American Academy for Emergency Psychiatry has developed core training competencies and guidelines for psychiatric residents and will be a key organization for the continued growth and development of the subspecialty of emergency psychiatry.

EMERGENCY PSYCHIATRY

PART I

Introduction to Principles of Emergency Psychiatry

Chapter 1

EMERGENCY MEDICINE APPROACH TO PSYCHIATRIC ILLNESS

INTRODUCTION

Psychiatric illness is prevalent in emergency departments. Patients are brought in voluntarily, by themselves or family members, or involuntarily, by the police or emergency medical services of the community, for evaluation of bizarre behaviors. As emergency physicians it is imperative to differentiate functional from organic symptoms. The disposition of a patient with a change in behavior from his norm hinges on the ability of the treating emergency physician to accurately determine which patient requires a medical intervention from one who requires emergent or urgent psychiatric care.

Ingestion of toxic substances and overdose of medication can lead to medical syndromes that must be recognized and treated prior to psychiatric consultation. Despite much toxic ingestion that occurs daily, specific treatment exists in only a few specific cases. These anti-dotes will be reviewed along with the supportive therapy that is appropriate for most ingestions.

Despite the high incidence of psychiatric illness in emergency departments, the emergency physician can manage the majority of these patients. Immediate psychiatric care is necessary for only the patients who represent a significant risk to life or limb.

The goals of this chapter include:

1. Review the common psychiatric manifestations of medical illness
2. Review the common medical manifestations of psychiatric illness
3. Review the common toxidromes of ingestions in table format, including common toxins and treatment
4. Review an algorithm of appropriate consultation of psychiatrists from the emergency department

PSYCHIATRIC MANIFESTATIONS OF MEDICAL ILLNESS

Psychiatric symptoms are common in the emergency department. Personality disorders, mood disorders, and frank psychosis frequently present for initial evaluation and treatment. A 1978 publication found a medical cause for psychiatric symptoms in 9.1% of psychiatric patients (Hall, 1978). These patients may have a primary psychiatric disorder with a coexisting medical condition, psychiatric symptoms secondary to their medical illness, or be exhibiting a psychiatric syndrome as a primary manifestation of their medical disorder. Adding intoxications with medications and recreational drugs into this mix of patients makes them even more complicated. This group of patients requires a thorough evaluation by a physician with a broad knowledge base in order to discern between the medical and psychological causes of disease.

The *Diagnostic and Statistical Manual of Mental Disorders,* 4th edition (1994) (DSM-IV) defines a psychiatric presentation of a medical illness as a "mental disorder due to a general medical condition. This is characterized as the presence of mental symptoms that are judged to be the direct physiological consequence of a general medical condition."

There are typical patterns of presentation for organic disease as outlined in Table 1-1. These features of illness that indicate an organic basis for disease are organized by the typical approach to a patient encounter. Being alert to the typical features of organic disease for each step in the patient care algorithm gives an improved ability to discover an organic basis for mental symptoms. Table 1-2 is a nonexhaustive list of the common features of organic disease organized by the primary psychiatric symptom.

TABLE 1-1 FEATURES SUGGESTIVE OF GENERAL MEDICAL CONDITIONS

History of present illness	• Late age of onset of new behavior symptoms • Temporal relationship between the onset or exacerbation of symptoms and a medical illness • Nonauditory hallucinations (visual hallucinations, illusions, and distortions have been reported to be the best indicators of medical basis of disease) (Hall, 1978) • Sudden onset of psychosis or delirium • Features that are atypical for a specific psychiatric diagnosis • Greater severity of symptoms than expected for the psychiatric illness alone
Medications	• Prescription drugs with psychoactive properties (digoxin) • Centrally acting medications • Intoxication with, or withdrawal from, a drug or toxin with psychiatric manifestations (e.g., delirium or psychosis), or the presence of a characteristic toxidrome even in the absence of specific history
Family history	• No personal or family history of psychiatric illness
Physical examination	• Abnormal vital signs • Evidence of increased intracranial pressure • Autonomic dysfunction with a history of good premorbid function • Detailed neurological examination abnormalities • Mental status examination abnormalities

Laboratory findings	• Abnormalities of any of the following ordered as appropriate for each patient
	  –Complete blood count
	  –Electrolytes (including calcium, magnesium, phosphorus)
	  –Renal function
	  –Urinalysis
	  –Hepatic function
	  –Toxic screen
	  –Electrocardiogram
	  –Imaging studies
	  –Lumbar puncture

Treatment	• Resistance to treatment with psychoactive medications

TABLE 1-2 TYPES OF PSYCHIATRIC ILLNESS AND ASSOCIATED MEDICAL DISEASE STATES

Illness	Defining Factors	Causative Disease States
General organic mental syndromes	See Table 1-1	Vitamin deficiency (B_{12}) Dementia Wilson's disease Neurosyphilis Leukodystrophies Neurodegenerative disorders Chronic meningitis Heavy metal poisoning Infections (encephalitis, meningitis)
Psychosis	Normal function prior to illness Age greater than 40 and sudden onset suggest medical cause Hallucinations or delusions often present	Structural lesions (neoplasm, calcification) Biochemical or physiological disturbance Lupus cerebritis Temporal lobe epilepsy Medications/intoxicants
Mania	Elderly onset	Medications/intoxicants Frontal-lobe syndromes Multiple sclerosis Epilepsy Infection Wilson's disease Cerebrovascular syndromes
Delirium	Elderly patients	Almost always medical Medications/intoxicants
Depression	Elderly patients	Epilepsy Parkinson's disease Stroke Frontal-lobe syndromes Multiple sclerosis Cushing's disease Major organ failure Endocrine disorders Metabolic disorders Medications/drugs
Anxiety	If more than 35 years old and no clear psychological precipitant, medical cause should be suspected Prominent anxiety Panic attacks Obsession/compulsion	Endocrine disorders Metabolic disorders Stroke Parkinson's disease Cardiovascular (cardiomyopathies, angina, arrhythmia) Pulmonary (COPD, asthma, pulmonary embolism) Medications/intoxicants

MEDICAL MANAGEMENT OF COMMON TOXIDROMES

Overdose or intoxication is a leading cause for both medical and psychiatric emergency visits. The overlap of toxicology, suicide attempts, and psychiatric illness mandates that emergency physicians and psychiatrists be able to recognize a toxidrome and initiate treatment of toxin ingestion.

GENERAL INFORMATION

The American Association of Poison Control Centers (AAPCC) Toxic Exposure Surveillance System (TESS) (www.AAPCC.com) data are compiled yearly. This database reports the common intoxicants that are encountered by poison control centers in the United States. This database includes over 29 million human exposures with 2.1 million for the year 2000. This database is dependent on emergency departments or patients to report toxic exposure patients to a poison control center; it does not include all states but it still represents the most complete data available.

Human exposures have remained stable at just over 2 million per year since 1994. Children under the age of 6 are involved in 52.7% of the cases. However, of the 920 reported deaths only 20 (2.2%) involved children. Clearly, adults tend to have more lethal exposures. The vast majority of exposures were unintentional (85.9%) with 7.5% being classified as suicide attempt and 7.0% as therapeutic error. Ninety-four percent of adolescent deaths and 79% of adult deaths were intentional. Clinical effects (signs, symptoms, or laboratory abnormalities) were noted in 30.7% of cases, with 80.8% considered as related to the exposure. Seventy-eight percent of the cases were managed outside of a health care facility, usually at the site of the exposure.

The most common agents were (in order of most to least): analgesics, cleaning substances, cosmetics, foreign bodies, plants, cough and cold preparations, bites and envenomations, sedatives/hypnotics/antipsychotics, topical agents, pesticides, antidepressants, food products, alcohols, hydrocarbons, antihistamines, antimicro-

bials, and chemicals. In comparison, the agents with the largest number of deaths are analgesics, antidepressants, sedative/hypnotics/antipsychotics, stimulants/street drugs, cardiovascular drugs, alcohols, anticonvulsants, muscle relaxants, gases and fumes, chemicals, antihistamines, cleaning substances, automotive products, antimicrobials, pesticides, and hydrocarbons.

GENERAL APPROACH TO THE POISONED PATIENT

All patients who present for health care should have their airway, breathing, and circulation (ABCs) evaluated first. This is followed by the vital signs and then a thorough history and physical examination. Laboratory testing and imaging can then be ordered in a rational manner. When all of the data are then collected, a plan of treatment and intervention can be initiated. These ideal steps must be flexible as necessary for each specific patient encounter. All life threats must be addressed as soon as discovered and other urgent needs addressed prior to the full exam being completed. In practice, several steps in the patient encounter and evaluation occur simultaneously. Often decisions to institute treatment to the poisoned patient must be made prior to all of the data being available. Finally, all evaluations should be documented in a legible format; however, this paperwork should never be allowed to delay patient care or disposition.

The history of present illness should include:

- Type of agent ingested
- Time of ingestion
- Amount ingested
- Symptoms pre- and postingestion
- Time since symptoms began
- Circumstances of exposure

Patients present to emergency departments at various times after their ingestions are complete (Kulig et al., 1985). Most commonly, patients are evaluated 2–4 hours after ingestion. Theoretically, this is when they become symptomatic and desire reversal of the symptoms.

A thorough past medical history, a list of allergies, and a list of all medications/poisons in the house should be sought. If the patient is unable to provide this information, use all means at your disposal to ascertain the information. This may include the emergency medical service that transported the patient, family members, witnesses, and local police departments.

Physical examination should be focused and include an objective measure of mental status. This will allow for serial measurements of cognitive function and therefore toxin activity.

Laboratory studies are of limited value in the poisoned patient. Poisons rarely cause routine abnormalities of common lab values such as electrolytes and blood counts. It is well recognized that poisoned patients commonly do not accurately report the agent(s) they took. Also, multiple ingestions are common. Therefore, measurement of serum levels of agents with delayed toxicity or difficult-to-recognize or clinically silent early syndromes should be considered in all patients. For this reason an acetaminophen level and salicylate level should be considered in all patients.

Routine comprehensive toxic screen is not recommended. Before the development of the toxic screen, clinicians depended on the clinical signs of poisoning to diagnose patients. Clinicians must continue to recognize common toxidromes because treatment is frequently required before a toxic screen can be completed. Also, many common poisons are missed on a routine toxic screen. The poisons tested for by a toxic screen are highly institution variable. For example, the benzodiazepine class of drugs is very large and while diazepam may be easily detected by your laboratory lorazepam may not. In this case, reliance on a toxic screen in a patient with the benzodiazepine toxidrome could be misleading.

Table 1-3 lists common toxidromes. Knowledge of these symptoms can lead to early recognition and treatment of the poisoned patient. These clinical signs of poisoning are reliable indicators of ingestion and should correlate with the patient's history. Patients who remain asymptomatic and clinically stable despite massive ingestion histories are not at risk for delayed compromise, except in the case of drugs that "slow release" or have late toxicity.

TABLE 1-3   COMMON SYNDROMES

Class	Agent	Symptoms
Analgesics	Salicylates	Hyperventilation, flushing, hyperthermia, tinnitus, nausea, vomiting
	Acetaminophen	Abdominal pains, nausea, vomiting, anorexia, liver failure
Narcotic syndrome	Heroin, morphine, codeine, meperidine	Miosis, decreased respirations, hypotension, coma
Cholinergic syndrome	Organophosphates, carbamates	Bradycardia, constricted pupils, salivation, lacrimation, bronchorrhea, defecation
Anticholinergic syndrome	Atropine, scopolamine, diphenhydramine	Tachycardia, dilated pupils, fever, agitation, delirium, dry skin, dry mucous membranes
Sedative hypnotic agents	Benzodiazepines	Coma, normal blood pressure, normal pulse, decreased reflexes
	Barbiturates	Decreased mental status, coma, hypotension, decreased respiration, blisters, hypothermia
	Nonbarbiturates	Fluctuating coma, decreased reflexes, decreased respirations, hypothermia
Antidepressants	Lithium	Decreased mental status, hyperreflexia, nausea, vomiting, polyuria, seizures, coma, tremor
	Monoamine oxidase inhibitors	Delayed toxicity, hypertension, muscular rigidity, hyperthermia
	Cyclic antidepressants	Decreased mental status, tachycardia, hyper-reflexia, cardiac conduction delays, seizures
Cardiovascular	Digoxin	Atrioventricular block, bradycardia, arrhythmia, delirium, hallucinations, visual disturbance, nausea, vomiting, confusions
	Beta blockers	Bradycardia, refractory hypotension, bronchspasm, congestive heart failure
	Calcium channel blockers	Hypotension, bradycardia, atrioventricular block, congestive heart failure

TREATMENT OF ACUTE POISONING

The majority of poisoned patients require only supportive care. Treatment consists of airway, breathing, and circulatory support along with decontamination and antidote administration. With the advent of ventilators, pharmaceutical management of blood pressure, dialysis, hemoperfusion, cardiac monitors, portable electroencephalographs, and other associated equipment we rarely witness a physiological compromise that cannot be treated.

Decontamination of the poisoned patient has traditionally included gastric emptying through emesis or lavage, cathartic agents, and activated charcoal delivery. These interventions have come under close scrutiny recently in an attempt to define a patient population that will benefit from these invasive, uncomfortable, and potentially harmful procedures.

A recent "State of the Art" review concluded that routine use of gastric lavage and administration of activated charcoal lead to a high rate of intubation, aspiration, and ICU admission. Therefore, gastric emptying in addition to activated charcoal cannot be considered the routine approach to patients. Most patients arrive at the emergency department 2 hours or more after their ingestion. This is long after the toxin has left the stomach and absorption has taken place. Activated charcoal is recommended if the patient:

- Arrives within 1–2 hours of ingestion, or
- Has ingested an agent that delays gastric motility, or
- The agent has delayed absorption.

But not if:

- The agent and quantity is known to be nontoxic, or
- The agent is not absorbed by activated charcoal (Bond, 2002).

Gastric lavage should not be undertaken unless the patient has ingested a potentially life-threatening amount of poison and the procedure can be undertaken within 60 minutes of ingestion. Even then, clinical benefit has not been confirmed in controlled studies (Vale, 1997).

Antidotes and specific treatments are available for a limited number of poisonous exposures. Several are commonly used (i.e., naloxone) while most are used infrequently and some are rarely used (i.e., d-penicillamine) or are not available in some areas of the country (i.e., crotalid antivenom).

Table 1-4 lists known antidotes, doses, and associated toxins. Patients who require an antidote administration require admission to a medical ward or intensive care unit and inpatient medical and psychiatric evaluation.

It is important to reemphasize that routine comprehensive toxicology testing does not screen for the majority of the agents for which antidotes are available. Therefore, most of these treatments are given based on history and clinical suspicion.

Delayed toxicity is a rare event. The only reported events of truly delayed toxicity are attributed to *Amanita* mushrooms and monoamine oxidase inhibitors (Linden et al., 1984; Olson et al., 1982). Ingestion of sustained-release tablets and enteric-coated preparations can lead to some delay of toxicity. How much of a delay is not known.

An observation period of 6 hours is generally adequate to observe for signs of toxicity. A patient who is asymptomatic, has a normal acetaminophen and salicylate level, and has a normal physical exam 6 hours after exposure is generally considered "medically cleared" for psychiatric evaluation. Patients with abnormal vital signs, symptoms of intoxication, or decreased mental status should be admitted for observation and treatment.

TABLE 1-4 TOXINS AND ANTIDOTES

Toxin	Antidote	Dose
Acetaminophen	*N*-Acetylcysteine	140 mg/kg PO load then 70 mg/kg q4hr for 17 doses
Narcotics (short acting)	Naloxone	0.4–2 mg SC/IV q2–3 min
Narcotics (long acting)	Naltrexone Nalmafene	50 mg PO qd 1–5 mg IV q4–8 hr.
Convulsants	Benzodiazepines	Drug dependent, for example; lorazepam 0.5–2 mg IM/IV q5min
Benzodiazepines	Flumazenil	0.2 mg IV q1min prn maximum of 5 doses per series or 3 mg/hr
Hypoglycemic agents, insulin	Glucose	D50 1 amp IV boluses and infusion to maintain glucose over 80 mg/dL
Hydrofluoric acid	Calcium gluconate	10% solution subQ Gel of 2.5% applied to burn Severe burns may require intra-arterial treatment
Hyperkalemia	Calcium chloride	500–1000 mg IV q10min prn
Snake and spider bites	Antivenin	Depends on severity of bite; Arizona poison control center (602)-626-6016
Cholinergic syndrome (i.e., organophosphates, nerve agents)	Atropine	2–4 mg IV q5–10min Titrate to drying of secretions
Alcohols	Ethanol	Oral: load with 0.8 mL/kg 95% ethanol, then 0.15 mL/kg/hr, IV: load with 7.6 mL/kg 10% ethanol over 1 hr, then 1.4 mL/kg/hr; maintain serum level 100–150 ng/dL
Hypoglycemia, Beta-blocker	Glucagon	1–5 mg IV/IM up to 10 mg
Warfarin	Phytonadione (vitamin K)	0.5–10 mg SC/IM/IV × 1 based on INR value
Digoxin	Fab fragments	# of 40-mg vials = (digoxin conc. [ng/mL] × weight [kg]) or (mg digoxin ingested × 1.33)
Methanol and ethylene glycol	Fomepizole	Load with 15 mg/kg IV then 10–20 mg/kg IV q12hr
Cyanide	Hydroxycobalamin (vitamin B_{12}) (investigational)	4 g IVP

(continued)

TABLE 1-4   TOXINS AND ANTIDOTES—Continued

Toxin	Antidote	Dose
Cyanide *(cont.)*	Lily antidote kit • Sodium thiosulfate • Sodium nitrite • Amyl nitrite	12.5 g IV 300 mg IV over 3–5 min Peds: 6–10 mg/kg Crush pearl under nose
INH, ethylene glycol, *Gyromitra* mushrooms	Pyridoxine (vitamin B_6)	INH: 1 g/g of INH ingested Ethylene glycol: 100 mg/kg/dose
Hyperglycemia, hyperkalemia	Insulin	Dosing varies Hyperglycemia: 0.1 U/kg/hr IV Hyperkalemia: 5–10 units IV
Carbon monoxide	Hyperbaric oxygen	Consult hyperbaric physician
Methanol, methotrexate	Folic acid	50–70 mg IV q4hr × 24 hr
Anticholinergic syndrome (atropine, scopolamine)	Physostigmine	0.5–1 mg SLOW IVP, max. 2 mg Have atropine immediately available
Lead (level > 45 μg/dL)	Succimer	10 mg/kg q8hr for 5 days, then 10 mg/kg q12hr for 14 days (approved only for pediatric usage)
Organophosphate, carbamates	Pralidoxime (2-PAM)	1–2 g IV over 15–30 min, may repeat once
Iron	Deferoxamine	15 mg/kg/hr IV
Methemoglobinemia	Methylene blue	1–2 mg/kg IV over 5 min (1% soln)
Heavy metal, radioisotope, and iron	EDTA	75 mg/kg/day divided in 3–6 doses for up to 5 days
Heavy metal poisoning	Dimercaprol (BAL) d-Penicillamine	2.5–5.0 mg/kg deep IM initial dose 25 mg/kg q6 mg PO daily
Wernicke's encephalopathy	Thiamine	100 mg IV/IM q day
Salicylates, cyclic antidepressants, amantidine, class 1 antidysrhythmics, ethylene glycol, methanol, phenobarbital, chlorpropamide, methotrexate	Alkalinization	Sodium bicarbonate 1–2 mEq/kg IVP boluses Cyclic antidepressant: use if QRS > 100–200 mscec or if hypotension exists Keep serum pH normal

BIBLIOGRAPHY

American Association of Poison Control Centers (AAPCC). http://www.AAPCC.com.

Bond GR. The Role of Activated Charcoal and Gastric Emptying in Gastric Decontamination: A State-of-the-Art-Review. *Annals of Emergency Medicine* 39 (March 2002): 273–86.

Diagnostic and Statistical Manual of Mental Disorders, 4th ed. (DSM-IV). Washington, DC: American Psychiatric Association, 1994.

Hall RCW, Popkin MK, DeVaul R, et al. Physical Illness Presenting as Psychiatric Disease. *Archives of General Psychiatry* 35 (1978): 1315–20.

Kulig K, Bar-or D, Cantrill SV, et al. Management of Acutely Poisoned Patients without Gastric Emptying. *Annals of Emergency Medicine* 14(6) (June 1985): 562–67.

Linden CH, Rumack BH, Schmitz B. Monoamine Oxidase Inhibitor Overdose. *Annals of Emergency Medicine* 13(12) (December 1984): 1137–44.

Olson KR, Pond SM, Seward J, et al. Amanita Phalloides, Type Mushroom Poisoning. *Western Journal of Medicine* 137 (1982): 282–89.

Vale JA. Position Statement: Gastric Lavage. American Academy of Clinical Toxicology; European Association of Poisons Centres and Clinical Toxicologists. *Journal of Toxicology—Clinical Toxicology* 35(7) (1997): 711–19.

Chapter 2

DIAGNOSTIC PRINCIPLES OF EMERGENCY PSYCHIATRY

INTRODUCTION

Diagnostic assessment in emergency psychiatric settings involves assessment of:

1. Whether the patient poses an acute risk to the examiner or to others in the treatment environment
2. Whether or not the patient is an appropriate subject for involuntary commitment
3. Whether the patient is suffering from an emergency medical or surgical problem
4. What treatment, if any, is necessary in the emergency setting
5. What referral is appropriate for the patient, particularly whether or not inpatient treatment is required
6. What preliminary psychiatric diagnoses should be made

These diagnostic assessments require:

1. A careful history from the patient, usually focusing on the history of the present illness
2. A mental status examination
3. Vital signs and, often, a physical examination and laboratory work
4. Collateral history from family and caregivers if possible

The goals of this chapter include:

1. Review the process for making an initial assessment of dangerousness of the patient to the interviewer and other staff and patients and review methods of assuring safety of the interviewers and others during the assessment process
2. Review the general process for interviewing patients in the emergency psychiatric setting and specify modifications of interview techniques for specific clinical problems
3. Discuss the emergency mental status examination
4. Discuss the emergency psychiatric physical assessment
5. Discuss appropriate use of laboratory assessment in emergency psychiatry
6. Review how to obtain and interpret history from medical records, family, and caregivers
7. Describe the decision process for involuntary commitment
8. Describe the decision process for hospitalization or release
9. Describe the decision process for community referral
10. Describe the process for making psychiatric diagnoses in the emergency setting

ASSURING A SAFE ENVIRONMENT FOR EMERGENCY EVALUATION

Emergency psychiatric evaluations often involve acutely agitated or, at least, upset patients with whom the examiner is not well acquainted. Staff injuries are, unfortunately, a continual risk in emergency psychiatry. Before doing anything else with the patient, the examiner must assure, as much as possible, his safety and that of the staff and patients in the environment.

In order to assure safety, the space for emergency psychiatric evaluation should provide:

1. Weapon screening
2. Rooms in which the examiner cannot be easily trapped
3. A choice of open or enclosed interviewing areas
4. A way to call for help
5. Adequate personnel to respond if help is needed, including trained security personnel

If a patient is brought in handcuffed by the police with a history of very recent assault, it may be necessary to examine this patient in physical restraints. If a patient is acutely agitated and threatening, it may be necessary to have security personnel physically standing by while the patient is interviewed. Every patient should be screened for weapons before being interviewed using a manual search and/or a handheld metal detector.

Patients should be regarded as a high risk for violence if they are:

1. Acutely intoxicated
2. Acutely paranoid or enraged
3. Extremely tense or restless as indicated by pacing, loudness, increased startle reflex, or elevated motor tension

Patients with these signs should be given a lot of space, and approached slowly with a bland and pleasant demeanor. Direct eye contact on the examiner's part, which might be interpreted as aggressive, should be avoided. If it is necessary to withdraw from a patient, that should ordinarily be done without turning one's back on the patient and with as few abrupt movements as possible.

INTERVIEWING IN THE PSYCHIATRIC EMERGENCY SETTING (TABLE 2-1)

Patients seen in emergency psychiatric settings are nearly always upset about something. Patients should be allowed to start off the interview talking about what is worrying them the most. Start with an open-ended question like "What brings you here today?" This is usually a good idea, even if the patient has already seen a triage person who has written down a chief complaint such as "hearing voices." Allow the patient to talk for at least five minutes without interruption. This approach will allow the examiner to see how the patient's thoughts and affects are flowing and will also convey a feeling that the examiner cares about what the patient perceives to be the most important problem. For each problem the patient mentions one should start with open-ended questions (e.g., "Could you say more about feeling depressed?") and move to closed-ended questions (e.g., "Have you been having trouble sleeping?").

Focus on helping the patient establish a chronology of his complaints. This, in itself, is often helpful to patients who are feeling overwhelmed and confused. Ask for a specific example rather than letting the patient stay vague in general (e.g., "About how many hours have you been sleeping the last few days?" or "What are some specific things that you have been feeling guilty about?"). Pay special attention to the question of why the patient is seeking treatment now rather than, say, next week. Try to delineate the patient's current level of symptoms and functioning compared to his or her "baseline," or typical, level of symptoms and functioning.

History of present illness and current social history are more important than past medical history or past social history. Generally, for an emergency evaluation patient, it is adequate to ascertain that a patient has a "long history of multiple psychiatric hospitalizations," rather than to define the exact dates of the hospitalizations. Past medical history for physical problems may be more important than in most psychiatric interviews because medical problems may be causing psychiatric symptoms and because many psychiatric patients may have been neglecting their medical care. Assess the patient's expectations for treatment (e.g., is the patient expecting to be hospitalized?).

The interview should be regarded as a therapeutic opportunity. Patients coming to emergency psychiatry frequently have a dangerously low level of self-esteem and it is important to try to help them leave the emergency room setting feeling better about themselves and their situation than they did when they came in. Reassurance should be given more freely than in other psychiatric settings and long silences should generally be avoided.

TABLE 2-1 PSYCHIATRIC HISTORY ELEMENTS FOR EMERGENCY EVALUATION

Patient identification
• Age, sex, marital status, insurance status, source of referral (e.g., self, police)

Chief complaint

History of present illness
• Symptoms
• Chronology of symptoms
• Current treatment
• Current living situation and social supports

Past psychiatric history
• Previous hospitalizations
• Previous diagnoses
• Previous medication
• Medical illnesses and treatment

Social history
• Educational (occupational/military)
• Marital

Family history of psychiatric illness

MENTAL STATUS EXAMINATION IN EMERGENCY PSYCHIATRY

A mental status examination should be recorded for every emergency psychiatric evaluation. Most of the material recorded for the mental status examination during the observational portion is assessed while gathering the history (see Table 2-2). It is particulary important to record that suicidal and homicidal ideation was assessed. The most common liability in the emergency psychiatric setting is failure to hospitalize patients needing involuntary hospitalization for risk of violence to self and/or others. Always remember that liability does not arise from being wrong in an assessment, but from being negligent in an assessment. If there is no evidence that dangerousness has been assessed, there is more liability risk than if risk has been assessed as present but the overall situation dictated release rather than hospitalization.

It is not necessary to do a formal psychometric mental status exam on every emergency psychiatric patient. If there is any question of possible contribution of general medical condition, orientation to time, place, and person should be assessed as should memory, immediate, recent, and remote. Serial sevens (e.g., "Start with 100, take away 7, and then take away 7 from the results") may be useful, or more often serial threes may be useful, as may questions of general information (e.g., "Who is the president of the United States?").

TABLE 2-2   **MENTAL STATUS ELEMENTS FOR EMERGENCY EVALUATION**

Observational portion
- Appearance, behavior, and attitude
- Mood and affect
- Speech and organization
- Thought content
- Suicide ideation
- Homicidal or violent ideation
- Hallucinations and delusions

Psychometric portion
- Cognitive function
- Level of consciousness
- Orientation
- Memory
- Attention and concentration
- Higher cortical functions

PHYSICAL ASSESSMENT

Every patient who needs an emergency psychiatric assessment certainly needs a physical assessment. Every patient who needs an emergency psychiatric assessment certainly does not need "a complete physical exam." Emergency medical practice includes a focused physical assessment but never an exhaustive physical assessment. Emergency psychiatric practice should be the same. Every patient who is seen as a psychiatric emergency needs:

1. Vital signs
2. A medically oriented inspection
3. A brief screening history

A patient does not ordinarily need a physical exam if he or she:

1. Has normal vital signs
2. Does not have a medical complaint
3. Is not delirious or demented
4. Does not have a history of chronic physical illness (e.g., diabetes)
5. Does not "look sick" (e.g., no signs of physical trauma, normal skin tone and color, normal respiration, normal posture and movement)

Whenever in doubt, it is, of course, appropriate to do a screening physical examination. If there is a medical emergency department in proximity, it is generally better to let the emergency medicine physicians do the physical exam because they do them more often than psychiatrists. From a medicolegal point of view the standard of care would generally be interpreted as favoring an exam by an emergency medicine physician rather than an emergency psychiatry physician, if such help were readily available. If such backup is not available, a physical examination by a psychiatrist is usually adequate to assess if referral for more extensive physical exam is necessary. The physical conditions that necessitate true emergency medical intervention are usually so severe that they can be picked up by a physician who does not do physical examinations very frequently.

There used to be a school of thought that psychiatrists should not do physical examinations because doing them would disturb the psychotherapeutic relationship with the patient. Such an attitude is no longer prevalent and is not at all appropriate in emergency psychiatry. The physical exam should, of course, not include genital, pelvic, or rectal exams. If there are concerns involving those parts of the anatomy, the patient should be referred to emergency medicine. Generally, patients respond positively to screening neurological and general medical exams by the psychiatrist. In many cases, patients, especially with first episodes of illness, are trying to make sense of a frightening and unfamiliar situation and are concerned on some level that they may have an undiagnosed medical condition.

LABORATORY TESTS AND X-RAYS

Complete blood counts, electrolytes, and liver function tests are almost always available in the emergency setting and results are ordinarily available quickly enough to be useful in emergency decision making (i.e., within about an hour). Such tests should be regarded as an extension of the physical exam rather than a substitute for it. Tests, such as thyroid functions, that will not be finished in an hour or so are not useful for emergency decision making and if they are ordered, a mechanism must be in place to follow up on them and communicate the results back to the patient. If x-rays may be indicated, it is probably better to refer the patient to the medical emergency room for evaluation.

Toxicological screens are frequently ordered in emergency psychiatric settings, and may be very helpful. Most hospitals have a routine stimulant screen available whose results may be returned in an hour or two and may help to determine whether the patient's acute symptoms are due to substance abuse or mental illness. Similarly, Breathalyzer or blood alcohol levels can be very helpful. Comprehensive toxicological screens, which check for 100 or more drugs, do not ordinarily yield results that are available to the emergency room, but may be ordered to provide guidance to the ongoing caregivers to the patient.

HISTORY FROM OTHER SOURCES

The standard of care in emergency psychiatry requires the use of sources in addition to the patient. The medicolegal standard for decision making is whether the average competent practitioner would have made a similar decision based on what was known or should have been known to the treating physician. Information from the old records, from treating clinicians in the community, and from family and friends is considered information that should have been known. An attempt should always be made to access old records. If the patient consents, an attempt should almost always be made to contact community clinicians, and, if necessary, friends and family. If there is a question of involuntary commitment, community, clinics, and friends and family can ordinarily be contacted without the patient's consent, should their input be necessary to make an appropriate decision about involuntary hospitalization.

DECISION PROCESS FOR INVOLUNTARY HOSPITALIZATION

The most important assessment in psychiatric emergency settings is probably the assessment of whether or not the patient is an appropriate subject for involuntary treatment under the state's commitment statute. Each state has a slightly different statute, but all have a two-step process for hospitalization of patients who may be dangerous to themselves or others due to mental illness. In most states, police officers or physicians can file a statement of belief that the patient is dangerous, as defined in the state statute, and is mentally ill, as defined in state statute. In some states, another class of individuals, such as psychologists, probation officers, or health officers, can have patients brought in for evaluation. The second stage of the commitment process requires that the patient be transported to a psychiatric setting, often a psychiatric emergency setting, for a preliminary professional assessment, which will result in involuntary treatment. Details of this evaluation are presented elsewhere in this volume. The evaluation, however, must be completed in some prescribed time and must be based on all available data, and not solely on the patient's answer to the question of whether he or she is having suicidal or homicidal ideation.

DECISION TO HOSPITALIZE

This decision is second only to the decision about involuntary treatment in importance. If a patient does qualify for involuntary treatment, hospitalization is necessary in almost all cases. In most hospals, voluntary hospitalizations are outnumbered these days by involuntary hospitalizations, since insurers will try not to pay for hospitalization unless there is dangerousness. Most insurers do, on paper, make allowance for hospitalization in the case of failure of outpatient treatment. Insurance preauthorization is necessary from the emergency service before admission in almost all of these cases. Hospitalization has a cost to the patient, in terms of stigmatization, as well as in time and in money. Hospitalization should be avoided if it is at all possible to manage the patient safety in the community.

COMMUNITY REFERRAL

Most psychiatric emergency settings admit about a third of the patients and refer about two-thirds to community treatment. Almost all communities have a shortage of treatment capacity in some or all areas (e.g., mental illness, substance abuse, or mental retardation). Psychiatric emergency services need to know what resources are actually available in the community, as opposed to those available theoretically, but that do not in fact, accept referrals. Sometimes it is necessary to ask patients to return to the emergency room one or more times for follow-up, particularly if medication has been started. Referrals to homeless shelters are undesirable, but are sometimes the only alternative in urban areas.

PSYCHIATRIC DIAGNOSES

Precise psychiatric diagnoses in psychiatric emergency services are less important than appropriate dispositions. The appropriate dispositions are more related to the patient's current functioning than to the precise psychiatric diagnosis. Frequently, diagnoses from the emergency room end up being relatively nonspecific (e.g., psychotic disorder not otherwise specified). Definitive diagnosis usually waits for the definitive treatment setting to which the patient is referred from psychiatric emergency service.

Chapter 3

BIOLOGICAL TREATMENT PRINCIPLES

INTRODUCTION

One of the mainstays of treatment in emergency psychiatry is psychotropic medication. It is important to understand the various classes of psychotropic agents available and the factors involved in selecting an appropriate medication in the emergency situation at hand. Much of this chapter is adapted from *Postgraduate Medicine on the Treatment of Behavioral Emergencies* (May 2001), reprinted with permission from McGraw-Hill.

The goals of this chapter include:

1. Review the definition of a behavioral emergency and guidelines on treatment once nonintrusive measures have been unsuccessful
2. Distinguish treatment from chemical restraint
3. Delineate factors involved in the choice of a medication for acute and severe behavioral dyscontrol (e.g., factors determining initial choice, PO vs. IM, diagnostic considerations)
4. Algorithms outlining first-line and second-line choices of PO vs. IM medications in various clinical situations (e.g., GMC vs. substance intoxication vs. primary psychiatric disturbance causing agitation unre-

sponsive to verbal and other less intrusive measures); treatment algorithms for agitation/behaviorial dyscontrol due to GMC, substance intoxication, primary psychiatric disturbance
5. Special populations (e.g., pregnant woman who is agitated, psychotic, unresponsive; violent and unmanageable child; agitated, aggressive patient with a complicating condition; frail, elderly patients on multiple medications)
6. Recommended strategies if inadequate response to medications given
7. Review of antipsychotic medications currently available with a table detailing specific prescribing information on each medication; side effects and drug–drug interactions including NMS, acute dystonic reactions—symptoms and management
8. Review of anti-EPS medications available
9. Review of antianxiety medications currently available with a table detailing specific prescribing information on each medication
10. Review of antidepressant medications currently available with a table detailing specific prescribing information on each medication
11. Review of mood stabilizing medications

currently available with a table detailing specific prescribing information on each medication

12. Risk management strategies

BEHAVIORAL EMERGENCY DEFINED

A constellation of symptoms may constitute a behavioral emergency including:

- Direct threat or assault
- Refusal to cooperate, intense staring
- Motor restlessness
- Purposeless movements
- Affective lability
- Loud speech
- Irritability
- Intimidating behavior
- Aggression to property
- Demeaning or hostile verbal behavior

As reviewed in other chapters (e.g., Chapter 8, "The Potentially Violent Patient"), it is advised that efforts be made to decrease these symptoms beginning with the least paternalistic or aggressive approaches first, e.g., approaching the patient calmly, offering food, beverage, or other assistance, offering voluntary medication to help the patient feel calmer. Safety for all involved—patient, other patients in the setting, staff—is the first priority in an emergency setting. If verbal strategies do not work, it is important to swiftly move to show of force and then to use of emergency medication and/or seclusion and restraint.

TREATMENT VS. CHEMICAL RESTRAINT

Treatment is defined as an intervention that follows from an assessment of a patient and a plan of care intended to improve the patient's underlying condition. A plan of care is determined in an emergency setting by a brief assessment (usually unstructured visual "eyeballing," although some clinicians use more structured checklists) conducted by the attending or resident psychiatrist sufficient to place the patient in an initial diagnostic category (e.g., psychotic or substance abuse). The diagnostic category then dictates a plan of care, which may include medications to target identified symptoms. Thus, medication used to treat a specific psychiatric diagnosis is treatment, not chemical restraint.

For this reason as well as others, the authors disagree with the use of droperidol, which had been recommended in a recent Expert Consensus Guideline on the treatment of behavioral emergencies. Droperidol is not a medication typically used in the treatment of any psychiatric diagnosis so its use is a chemical restraint by definition (i.e., CMS [Center of Medicaid and Medicare Services, formerly HCFA] interim final rules dictate that a medication must be prescribed as a part of a plan of care to be considered treatment). Droperidol was taken off the European market because it has a negative cardiac effect (prolongation of QT interval), is not available in PO form, and has a fast onset and a fast offset.

USE OF MEDICATION IN BEHAVIORAL EMERGENCIES

The clinician has determined that the patient cannot respond to less intrusive interventions such as verbal de-escalation, the offering of food/beverage, or voluntary oral medications. In a patient determined to be uncooperative, agitated, confused, nondirectable, and exhibiting other behaviors delineated in the definition of behavioral emergency, the authors recommend the following steps for safe management.

1. Step one. Make an effort to:
   - Rule out drug allergies
   - Rule out drug adverse reactions
   - Rule out GMCs
   - Rule out medical contraindications to medication
   - Review prior treatment records
   - Rule out substance abuse
   - Determine history of positive medication responses
   - Determine if patient has a medication preference
2. Step two. The initial choice of medication depends on:
   - Speed of onset
   - Reliability of preparation
   - IM preparation
   - Duration of action
   - Side effect profile
   - Past patient response
   - Patient preference
   - Availability of liquid form of medication

   In a fast-paced emergency department, decisions are made swiftly with safety of all involved being the number one consideration. This is why speed of onset and IM preparation availability are so crucial. The emergency psychiatrist is secondarily concerned about long-term compliance and the availability of a depot medication for those patients with chronic nontreatment adherence.

   There are situations when it is best to avoid IM medications. These include:

   - Risk of side effects
   - Mental or emotional trauma to the patient
   - Compromising the clinician–patient relationship
   - Physical trauma
   - Exposure to contaminated needles
   - Effects of long-term medication adherence
3. Step three. Medication choices based on etiology:
   a. A behavioral emergency, (e.g., agitation determined to be due to a primary psychiatric disturbance requires swift and appropriate treatment in order to maintain the patient's safety as well as the safety and protection of others in the treatment environment) (Figure 3-1).

   It is often appropriate to load a patient experiencing a manic or mixed or dysphoric episode with Divalproex, particularly if:
   - The patient has a history of a positive response to Divalproex
   - Liver function tests are normal
   - Patient and family wish to avoid a hospitalization
   - Recommended dosing strategies for Divalproex:
     –Initiate at 20 mg/kg and continue until blood levels are available *or*
     –Loading dose: 30 mg/kg for 2 days, followed by 20 mg/kg beginning on day 3
   b. Often patients who are under the influence of substances become agitated and uncooperative, often posing an immediate risk of danger to themselves and/or others. Within the first hour of presentation with such a behavioral emergency, the following algorithm is advised (Figure 3-2).
   c. Often patients will present with complicating conditions such as comorbid medical conditions. The algorithm in Figure 3-3 addresses behavioral agitation that is due to, or complicated by, other medical conditions.

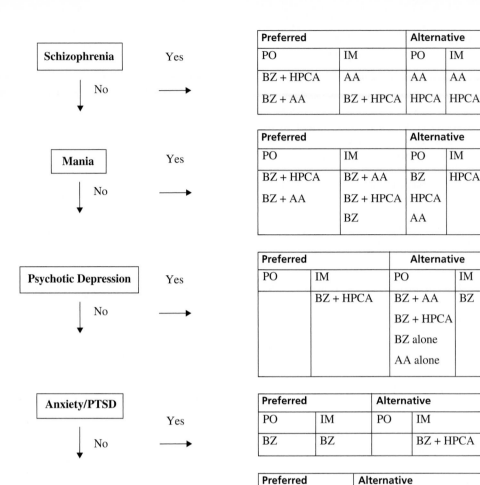

Schizophrenia — Yes

Preferred		Alternative	
PO	IM	PO	IM
BZ + HPCA	AA	AA	AA
BZ + AA	BZ + HPCA	HPCA	HPCA

No →

Mania — Yes

Preferred		Alternative	
PO	IM	PO	IM
BZ + HPCA	BZ + AA	BZ	HPCA
BZ + AA	BZ + HPCA	HPCA	
	BZ	AA	

No →

Psychotic Depression — Yes

Preferred		Alternative	
PO	IM	PO	IM
	BZ + HPCA	BZ + AA	BZ
		BZ + HPCA	
		BZ alone	
		AA alone	

No →

Anxiety/PTSD — Yes

Preferred		Alternative	
PO	IM	PO	IM
BZ	BZ		BZ + HPCA

No →

Personality Disorder No data — Yes

Preferred		Alternative	
PO	IM	PO	IM
		BZ	BZ alone
			BZ + HPCA

Figure 3-1 *Agitation due to primary psychiatric diagnosis.*

Source: Allen MH, et al. The Expert Consensus Scale. In Treatment of Behavioral Emergencies. *Postgraduate Medicine* (May 2001) (hereafter Allen et al. 2001).

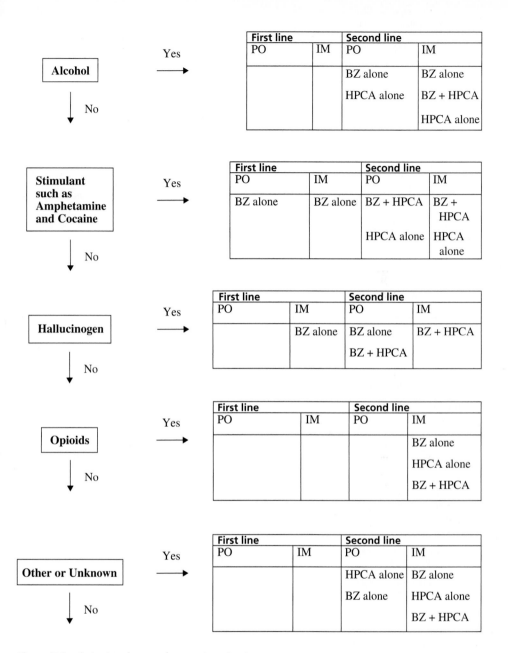

Figure 3-2 *Agitation due to substance intoxication.*

SOURCE: Allen et al. (2001). Reprinted with permission from McGraw-Hill.

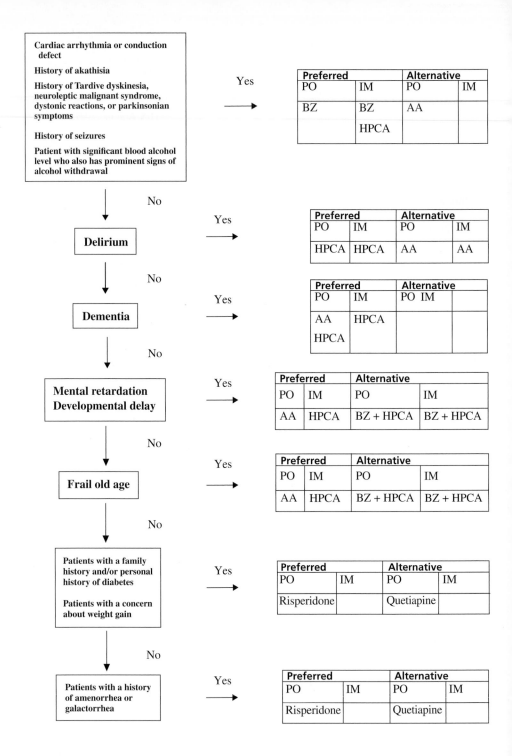

Figure 3-3 *Agitation due to or complicated by a general medical condition.*

SOURCE: Allen et al. (2001). Reprinted with permission from McGraw-Hill.

STRATEGIES IF INADEQUATE RESPONSE TO INITIAL INTERVENTIONS

Knowing when to change medication strategies in a patient who is not responding or only expe-riencing a partial response is important. First, be sure to allow sufficient time for the medica-tion to take effect. If after 45–60 minutes there has been no appreciable change or partial response, consult Table 3-1.

TABLE 3-1 **AGITATION IN SPECIAL POPULATIONS**

	Preferred	Alternative
Frail elderly	AA	HPCA
Children/adolescents*		Low-dose BZ
		Antihistamine
Pregnant females†	HPCA	AA
Mentally retarded/developmentally delayed		AA

*For a violent and unmanageable child.
†For a pregnant woman who is agitated, psychotic, and unresponsive to direction.

SOURCE: Allen et al. (2001). Reprinted with permission from McGraw-Hill.

REVIEW OF ANTIPSYCHOTIC MEDICATIONS (TABLES 3-2 TO 3-5)

ANTIPSYCHOTIC VS. NEUROLEPTIC VS. PHENOTHIAZINE

TERMINOLOGY CLARIFIED Neuroleptic is an older term meaning something that "seizes the nervous system." This was based on the belief that only those medications that caused extrapyramidal symptoms were effective antipsychotics.

Antipsychotic is the preferred and more accurate term. Phenothiazine refers to just one class of antipsychotic agents, e.g., chlorpromazine). There are a number of other classes such as thioxanthenes, butyrophenones, dibenzoxazepines, etc.

The indications for antipsychotic medications are many, but the primary focus of this chapter is to guide the clinician in making appropriate medication choices in particular for patients who are experiencing behavioral agitation, aggression, or other signs and symptoms of a behavioral emergency that requires treatment with psychotropic medication. Mechanisms of action are beyond the scope of this concise guide. Indications for the use of antipsychotic medication include the following, although the list is not exhaustive:

- Psychosis
- Schizophrenia
- Schizoaffective disorder
- Schizophreniform disorder
- Delusional disorder
- Brief psychotic disorder
- Bipolar disorder
- MDD with psychotic features
- Tourette's disorder
- OCD
- BPD
- MR/DD
- Secondary Psychotic states:
  Due to GMC (i.e., AIDS, delirium)
  Due to substance use

Of concern at the time of the writing of this book are weight gain and type II DM associated with atypical antipsychotic medication. Certainly there is much to recommend them including:

- Improved negative symptoms
- Improved positive symptoms
- Better side effect profile
- Improved cognition
- Less TD risk

Neuroleptic malignant syndrome (Table 3-6) is a particularly alarming potential side effect of anitpsychotic agents presumably caused by blockade of the dopaminergic pathways in the basal ganglia and hypothalamus and possibly from the sudden withdrawal of a dopamine agonist.

TABLE 3-2 **CONVENTIONAL ANTIPSYCHOTIC MEDICATION**

Generic Name	Trade Name	PO Doses Available	IM Available	Dosage Range (mg/day)
Chlorpromazine	Thorazine	10, 25, 50, 100, 200 30, 75, 150, 200, 300 sustained release	Yes	150–1000
Thioridazine	Mellaril	10, 15, 25, 50, 100, 150, 200,	No	100–800
Mesoridazine	Serentil	10, 25, 50, 100		75–300
Fluphenazine	Prolixin	1, 2.5, 5, 10	Yes	2–20
Perphenazine	Trilafon	2, 4, 8, 16	No	8–40
Trifluoperazine	Stelazine	1, 2, 5, 10	No	5–30
Thiothixene	Navane	1, 2, 5, 10, 20		6–50
Haloperidol	Haldol	0.5, 1, 2, 5, 10, 20	Yes	0.5–20

TABLE 3-3 **ATYPICAL ANTIPSYCHOTIC MEDICATION**

Generic Name	Trade Name	PO Doses Available	IM Available	Dosage Range (mg/day)
Risperidone	Respirdal	0.25, 0.5, 1, 2, 3, 4	No	1–6
Olanzapine	Zyprexa	2.5, 5, 7.5, 10, 15, 20	Soon	2.5–30
	Zydis	5,10		2.5–10
Quietiapine	Seroquel	25, 100, 200, 300	No	150–800
Ziprasidone	Geodon	20, 40, 60, 80	20 mg/ml	80–160
Clozapine	Clozaril	25, 100	No	200–1000
Aripripazole	Abilify	10, 15, 20, 30	No	10–30

TABLE 3-4 CONVENTIONAL ANTIPSYCHOTIC MEDICATION COMPARATIVE SIDE EFFECT PROFILE

Generic Name	Trade Name	Sedation	EPS	Anticholinergic	Orthostasis	Other Side Effects with Significant Incidence
Chlorpromazine	Thorazine	+++	+	+++	+++	
Thioridazine	Mellaril	+++	+	+++	+++	
Mesoridazine	Serentil	+++	+	++	++	
Fluphenazine	Prolixin	+	+++	+	+	
Perphenazine	Trilafon	+	++	+	++	
Trifluoperazine	Stelazine	+	+++	+	+	
Thiothixene	Navane	+	+++	+	+	
Haloperidol	Haldol	+	+++	+	+	

+++ = severe
++ = moderate
+ = mild
+/− = minimal

TABLE 3-5 ATYPICAL ANTIPSYCHOTIC MEDICATION COMPARATIVE SIDE EFFECT PROFILE

Generic Name	Trade Name	Sedation	EPS	Anticholinergic	Orthostasis	Other Side Effects with Significant Incidence
Risperidone	Respirdal	+	++	+	+	
Olanzapine	Zyprexa	++	+/−	+	+	Weight gain Drowsiness
Quietiapine	Seroquel	++	+/−	+	+	Drowsiness
Ziprasidone	Geodon	+	+/−	+	+/−	EKG changes
Clozapine	Clozaril	+++	+/−	++	+++	Seizure Agranulocytosis Drowsiness Weight gain

+++ = severe
++ = moderate
+ = mild
+/− = minimal

TABLE 3-6 NEUROLEPTIC MALIGNANT SYNDROME

Core Symptoms	Laboratory Findings	Management of NMS
Hyperthermia	Elevated CPK	Supportive measures such as stopping medication, hydration
Severe muscle rigidity, lead pipe	Elevated WBC	Dopamine agonists such as bromocriptine 5 mg tid
Diaphoresis	Elevated LFTs	Dantrolene
Delirium	Myoglobinuria	
Muteness		
Incontinence		
Rhabdomyolysis		
Mutism		
Autonomic instability		

REVIEW OF ANTICHOLINERGIC MEDICATIONS

Anticholinergic agents are indicated for the prevention of extrapyramidal side effects associated with antipsychotic medications (Table 3-7).

The main side effects associated with anticholinergic agents include:

- Dry mouth
- Blurry vision
- Constipation/bowel obstruction
- Confusional states

For the main drug interactions with anticholinergic agents, see Table 3-8.

TABLE 3-7 AGENTS FOR TREATMENT OF EXTRAPYRAMIDAL SIDE EFFECTS OF ANTIPSYCHOTIC MEDICATIONS

Generic Name	Trade Name	Usual Dosage (mg/day)
Amantadine	Symmetrel	100–200 bid
Benzotropine	Cogentin	0.5–2 bid; 1–2 mg IM for acute dystonic reaction
Biperiden	Akineton	2–6 tid; 2 mg IM
Clonazepam	Klonopin	0.5–1 bid
Diphenhydramine	Benadryl	25–50 bid; 25–50 IM for acute dystonic reaction
Procyclidine	Kemadrin	2.5–5 tid
Trihexyphenidyl	Artane, Tremin	2–5 tid

TABLE 3-8 ANTICHOLINERGIC DRUG INTERACTIONS

Medication/Drug Combined with Anticholinergic	Effect
Antipsychotic	Additive anticholinergic effect
Benzodiazepine	May increase cognitive impairment
TCA	Additive anticholinergic effect (e.g., dry mouth, urinary retention)

REVIEW OF ANTIANXIETY MEDICATIONS

Also known as anxiolytics and sedative-hypnotics, antianxiety medications (see Table 3-9) are chiefly made up of the drug class benzodiazepines. Others, such as antihistamines, beta-blockers, and the azapirone buspirone, will also be reviewed.

The indications for the use of these medications include:

- GAD
- Panic disorder
- Short-term stress-related insomnia
- Adjunctive treatment for mania
- Adjunctive treatment for psychosis
- Alcohol withdrawal
- EPS
- Nocturnal myoclonus
- Night terrors

Buspirone is indicted for the treatment of GAD, adjunctive treatment of OCD, dementia-related agitation, sexual dysfunction, and, in higher doses, as an antidepressant.

The side effects of anxiolytics and sedative-hypnotics are given in Table 3-10. Drug–drug interactions with antianxiety agents are given in Table 3-11.

TABLE 3-9 **ANTIANXIETY MEDICATIONS**

Generic Name	Trade Name	Dosages Available (mg)	Usual Daily Adult Dose (mg)
Alprazolam	Xananx	0.25, 0.5, 1,2	0.5–4*
Chlordiazepoxide	Librium	5, 10, 25	15–100
Clonazepam	Klonopin	0.5, 1, 2	0.5–4
Clorazepate	Tranxene	3.75, 7.5, 15 (11.25, 22.5 single-dose tablets)	15–60
Diazepam	Valium	2, 5, 10 15 mg sustained release	
Halazepam	Paxipam	20, 40	60–160
Lorazepam	Ativan	0.5, 1, 2	
Oxazepam	Serax	10, 15, 30	30–120
Prazepam	Centrax	5, 10, 20	20–60
Estazolam	ProSom	1, 2	
Flurazepam	Dalmane	15, 30	15–30
Quazepam	Doral	7.5, 15	7.5–15
Temazepam	Restoril	7.5, 15, 30	15–30
Triazolam	Halcion	0.125, 0.25	0.125–0.5*

*Do not exceed 0.25 in the elderly.

TABLE 3-10   SIDE EFFECTS OF ANXIOLYTICS/SEDATIVE-HYPNOTICS

Medication	Possible Effects
Benzodiazepines	Drowsiness
	Fatigue
	Weakness
	Light-headedness
	Ataxia
	Respiratory suppression
	Falls
	Confusion
	Psychomotor impairment
	Amnesia
	Depression
	Paradoxical excitement
	Psychological/physical dependence
Buspirone	Dizziness
	Gastrointestinal disturbance
	Headache
Antihistamines	Memory impairment/confusion

TABLE 3-11   DRUG–DRUG INTERACTIONS WITH ANTIANXIETY AGENTS

Medication Combined with Benzodiazepines	Effect
Cimetidine	May increase the plasma levels and toxicity of oxidatively metabolized BZs, i.e., long-acting BZs such as diazepam
Erythromycin	
Nefazadone	May increase plasma levels of triazolo-BZs
Rifampin	
Phenytoin	May decrease the clinical effect
Antacids	Slow absorption and decrease the clinical effect
Anticholinergic agents	Increase cognitive impairment
Clozapine	Increase sedation and respiratory suppression
Alcohol, narcotics, CNS depressants	BZs increase neurotoxicity of these agents; thus while BZs alone may have little toxicity in overdose, the combination with these agents may be lethal

Medications Combined with Buspirone	
SSRIs	Combinations may increase risk of serotonin syndrome
MAOIs	

REVIEW OF ANTIDEPRESSANT MEDICATIONS (TABLE 3-12)

Indications for the use of antidepressant medication include depressive disorders such as MDD, dysthymic disorder, anxiety disorders such as PTSD, panic disorder, OCD, social phobia, and eating disorders.

TABLE 3-12 **ANTIDEPRESSANT MEDICATIONS**

Generic Name	Trade Name	Dosages available (mg)	Usual daily adult dose (mg/day)
Amitriptiline	Elavil, Endep	10, 25, 50, 75, 100, 150	75–250
Amoxapine	Asendin	25, 50, 100, 150	200–300
Buproprion	Wellbutrin, Wellbutrin SR	100, 150	300
Citolapram	Celexa	20, 40	20–40
Clomipramine	Anafranil	25, 50, 75	50–200
Desipramine	Norpramin, Pertofrane	10, 25, 50, 75, 100, 150	75–250
Doxepin	Sinequan, Adapin	10, 25, 50, 75, 100	75–250
Fluoxetine	Prozac	10, 20	10–40
Fluvoxamine	Luvox	50, 100	50–250
Imipramine hydrochloride	Tofranil	10, 25, 50	75–250
Maprotiline	Ludiomil	25, 50, 75	50–200
Mirtazapine	Remeron	15, 30	15–45
Nefazadone	Serzone	100, 150, 200, 250	200–500
Nortriptiline	Aventyl, Pamelor	10, 25, 50, 75	50–100
Paroxetine	Paxil	10, 20, 30, 40	10–40
Protriptyoine	Vivactil	5, 10	20–45
Sertraline	Zoloft	50, 100	50–200
Trazadone	Desyrel	50, 100, 150, 300	50–400
Trimipramine	Surmontil	25, 50, 100	75–250
Venlafaxine	Effexor, Effexor SR	25, 37.5, 75, 100	75–300

REVIEW OF MOOD STABILIZING MEDICATIONS (TABLE 3-13)

TABLE 3-13 **MOOD STABILIZERS**

Generic Name	Brand Name	Capsules/ Tablets (mg)	Usual Daily Dose (mg/day)
Carbamazepine	Tegretol	100 (chewable) 200 (suspension, also available as 100 mg/5 mL)	400–800
Divalproex	Depakote Depakote Sprinkle	125, 250, 500 125	500–2000
Lithium carbonate	Eskalith	150, 300, 600	600–1500
Slow-release lithium carbonate	Lithobid	300	600–1500
	Eskalith CR	450	450–1350
Lithium citrate		8 meq/5 mL	Each 5 mL = 300 mg lithium carbonate
Gabapentin	Neurontin	200, 300, 400	200–800
Lamotrigine	Lamictal	25, 100, 150, 200 chewable 2, 5, 25	Target dose is 200 mg/day

RISK MANAGEMENT STRATEGIES

- Communicate with the ongoing therapist and/or treating psychiatrist/physician. Optimally, the physician working with the patient on an ongoing basis should always prescribe medication. When this is not possible, communication with the ongoing therapist is always indicated. When such communication is not possible, only small supplies of medication should be prescribed.
- If a patient is doing fairly well, do not change the medication. Even if the medication regimen is not what the emergency physician would choose, it should probably be continued and concerns communicated to the ongoing physician rather than attempting to change a long-term regimen on a short-term basis. An exception, of course, would be a case in which the emergency physician considers the ongoing medication to be so unacceptable as to constitute malpractice (e.g., long-term high-dose amphetamines for weight loss). In such a case, it would be unethical to continue the regimen.
- Be careful with medications that can be abused or that are medically dangerous when taken in overdose. Benzodiaepines and trycyclic antidepressants should ordinarily not be prescribed in more than 2-week quantities from an emergency service. For patients who are very suicidal or on very high doses, even a 1-week supply of tricyclics may be risky, in that 1 g of amitryptiline may be potentially fatal for a patient weighing 50 kg.
- Avoid prescribing narcotics. The physician treating the condition causing the pain should prescribe narcotics for pain. Narcotics for treatment of withdrawal should ordinarily be prescribed only at a licensed detoxification center. Refilling "lost" narcotic prescriptions almost always means prescribing drugs for abuse or resale on the streets. At the time of this writing, oxycontin is a particularly popular narcotic termed "hillbilly heroin."
- Discourage use of the emergency service as an alternative to ongoing treatment. It is acceptable to write prescriptions for patients from time to time when they have missed a clinic appointment, but not to do so repetitively.
- Do not expect much benefit acutely. It is widely recognized that most psychotropic agents do not have an immediate onset of action.
- Do not get too fancy. An emergency situation is not the situation for trying complicated or experimental regimens. Patients will have trouble adhering to them and physicians will have trouble evaluating the results.
- Ascertain what other medications the patient may be taking and which illnesses the patient may have. A medical history, and, in many cases, a physical examination, is called for before initiation of medication.
- Nonpharmacological interventions are generally preferable.
- Write out in longhand the number of units to be dispensed (e.g., Disp: #10 [ten]) to guard against prescription alteration.

BIBLIOGRAPHY

American Psychiatric Association. *Practice Guidelines for the Treatment of Psychiatric Disorders: Compendium 2002.* http://www. psych.org.

Chapter 4

PSYCHOSOCIAL PRINCIPLES

INTRODUCTION

This chapter reviews the psychological and social factors often involved in psychiatric emergencies and companion interventions that may be helpful in resolving the emergency situation successfully. The aim of this chapter is to give the clinician a psychosocial framework with which to understand each individual patient and to guide in formulation of clinically appropriate crisis resolution.

The Chinese character for crisis is a combination of two words—danger and opportunity. While few would choose to experience trauma in order to grow and transform, people often discover how resilient they are only in the face of crisis situations.

The goals of this chapter include:

1. Defining terms including biopsychosocial and psychosocial intervention
2. Defining typical means by which human beings maintain emotional equilibrium; defining and distinguishing defense mechanisms and coping strategies
3. Reviewing crisis intervention, active listening, and CALM mnemonic
4. Reviewing psychosocial algorithm summary
5. Reviewing risk management strategies

BIOPSYCHOSOCIAL MODEL

DEFINITION

The biopsychosocial model refers to the biological, psychological, and social factors that contribute to the etiology of a mental illness.

Biological refers to the individual's genetic predisposition, general medical conditions, and medications that may contribute to the etiology of a mental condition.

Psychological refers to the individual's charactistic defense mechanisms and coping strategies. An intervention might then be aimed in part at altering his coping style, shoring up or breaking down existing defense mechanisms, or helping to improve existing coping strategies (e.g., a person who tends to isolate and drink when experiencing stressors may be encouraged to stop drinking and attend Alcoholics Anonymous).

Social refers to the individual's family, school, peer relationships, interpersonal and occupational relationships, and their impact on his/her development. Understanding these factors lends itself to an intervention to increase supports that will be useful and utilized by the individual (e.g., a teenager arguing with her parents is close to her grandmother; thus one intervention might include a respite at her grandmother's home).

WHAT HAPPENS TO AN INDIVIDUAL EXPERIENCING A PSYCHIATRIC EMERGENCY?

Simply stated, an individual becomes overwhelmed by emotional conflicts and internal and/or external stressors and is unable to manage with his/her usual defense mechanisms/coping strategies.

Often there are myriad reasons why a person may experience a psychiatric emergency (e.g., psychosis, substance intoxication, loss or absence of an important supportive figure such as a case manager or a psychiatrist being on vacation, a parent's death, or a spouse/significant other's illness or job loss (Table 4-1).

There are a subset of individuals who utilize the emergency department to find housing and meals. Such "patients" may malinger psychiatric symptoms in an effort to meet basic survival needs. Often these are individuals who have burned bridges with many agencies in the community, making them doubly frustrating to assist. In Part II, the authors will address malingering as well as how to humanely handle these not infrequent situations.

TABLE 4-1 **EXAMPLES OF PSYCHOSOCIAL FACTORS THAT MAY CONTRIBUTE TO A PSYCHIATRIC EMERGENCY**

Poor coping strategies (e.g., isolating from others, substance abuse, gambling, and other addictive behaviors)

Change in family structure (e.g., getting married or divorced, blended families, births, an elderly relative moving in)

Change in friends, support group

Moves (e.g., from a parent's home to a group home; from a group home to independent living)

Losses, such as death, illness, job loss

Changes at work, school, day treatment program

Change in caregivers (e.g., case manager change, psychiatrist change)

COPING STRATEGIES AND DEFENSE MECHANISMS

Although defense mechanisms are also referred to as coping styles in the DSM-IV-TR, the authors disagree that they are necessarily the same. In the authors' view, coping styles or strategies are typically conscious choices to deal with emotional conflicts and internal or external stressors while defense mechanisms are largely automatic and unconscious mechanisms employed by the ego to defend against anxiety. Both share the goal of anxiety reduction.

COPING STRATEGIES

Examples of coping strategies are given in Table 4-2.

TABLE 4-2   **EXAMPLES OF COPING STRATEGIES**

Strategy	Healthy	Unhealthy
Task-focused behavior	x	
Emotional distancing		x
Cognitive self-talk	x	
Altruism	x	
Social—peer support	x	
Substance abuse		x
Addictive behaviors such as promiscuity, pathological gambling		x
Exercise/action (e.g., jogging, aerobics, walking)	x	
Relaxation exercises (e.g., stretching, yoga)	x	
Crying	x	
Humor	x	
Prayer/meditation	x	
Massage	x	
Music and art (e.g., creating and/ or appreciating)	x	
Adopt balanced diet and normalize sleep cycle	x	
Avoid overusing stimulants like caffeine, nicotine	x	
Write about the painful experience for yourself and to share with others	x	
Commit to something meaningful daily	x	

Note: Excessive employment may shift a healthy coping strategy into an unhealthy one (e.g., a husband and father spends all of his free time running to the detriment of occupational and familial roles and responsibilities).

DEFENSE MECHANISMS

The individual deals with emotional conflict, internal stressors, or external stressors via six different levels of defense mechanisms (Table 4-3).

TABLE 4-3 **DEFENSE MECHANISMS**

Level	Purpose/description	Examples
Highly adaptive	Maximizes gratification and allows conscious awareness of feelings, ideas, and their consequences, and promotes optimum balance among conflicting motives	Anticipation Affiliation Altruism Humor Self-assertion Self-observation Sublimation Suppression
Mental inhibitions, compromise formation (disavowal)	Keeps potentially threatening ideas, feelings, memories, wishes, or fears out of awareness with or without a misattribution of these to external causes	Denial Displacement Dissociation Intellectualization Isolation of affect Projection Rationalization Reaction formation Repression Undoing
Minor-image distorting	Distortions of image of self, body, or others employed to regulate self-esteem	Devaluation Idealization Omnipotence
Major-image distorting	Gross distortions or misattributions of image of self and others	Autistic fantasy Projective identification Splitting of self-image or image of others
Action	Deals with stressors by action or withdrawal	Acting out Apathetic withdrawal Help-rejecting complaining Passive-aggressive
Defensive dysregulation	Failure of defensive regulation to contain the individual's reaction to stressors, leading to a pronounced break with reality	Delusional projection Psychotic denial Psychotic distortion

CRISIS INTERVENTION

Once the clinician has a general framework for understanding patients, the clinician can proceed to understanding the individual patient and why he is presenting now in a crisis situation.

The goals of crisis intervention are:

- Establish rapport and trust
- Identify the precipitating stressor(s) that caused the crisis state
- Help the patient understand the meaning of the event
- Problem-solve together to resolve the crisis
- Provide referral information when appropriate

The ultimate goal of the emergency psychiatry intervention is to return emotional control to the patient and reestablish emotional equilibrium. The authors offer the CALM mnemonic to help clinicians remember the steps involved in crisis intervention.

C: Be CONCISE and specific; CLARIFY distortions.

Why is the patient presenting now? What are reasonable expectations in resolving this emergency?

A: ALLOW time for the person to process information.

Because of time constraints, it is necessary to continually refocus on the immediate emergent situation and options for how to best resolve it. Simultaneously, the clinician is soothing, reassuring, and helping the patient feel hopeful. Moreover, the clinician is conveying expertise, ability to help, and empathy all in a timely manner.

L: LISTEN using active listening skills; LISTEN for facts and feelings.

Active listening skills (Table 4-4) involve empathic listening for emotions that goes beyond the content or facts to listen to how the person feels. Empathy implies understanding and objectivity. The purpose of utilizing such skills is to:

- Facilitate rapport
- Encourage the patient to express himself and to accurately identify the problem(s)
- Show that the clinician is listening and understands both the facts and feelings
- Cull the important ideas, facts, feelings to establish the basis for further discussion and specifically problem solving

M: MAKE choices; empower the individual in crisis to review options and make choices.

Sometimes the greatest challenge to a busy clinician is redirecting the patient to a problem-solving mode as quickly and with as much diplomatic sensitivity as possible (e.g., "I am sorry for the pain you are feeling, I wish that we did have more time to talk now . . . I do think you are a person who would do well talking with a counselor or therapist about this . . . you are obviously verbal and insightful and want to talk about your feelings. What would you think about a referral to a therapist? If you like, we can review other options that might be helpful to you . . . I've got some other ideas about options for you . . . would you like to talk about them?").

Sometimes the individual needs time to process information. The clinician can review a couple of options, keep them simple, and leave the patient to think them over for a little while. Sometimes a help-rejecting patient will shoot down all of the options presented (e.g., a repeat alcohol abuser who is refusing AA referrals and insists that he doesn't have an alcohol problem; give him the opportunity to change his mind without losing face by indicating respectfully that should he change his mind, he is always welcome to call back for the information and "we will be happy to provide it"). If the patient is at imminent risk of harm to self or others, this of course triggers another threshold of clinical decision making that is covered thoroughly in other chapters (e.g., involuntary hospitalization).

TABLE 4-4 ACTIVE LISTENING SKILLS

Type	Example
Emotional labeling	Telling the person what emotion is heard in his/her voice (e.g., "You sound depressed"; "I am hearing anger in your voice")
Paraphrasing or restating	Repeating what the patient said in different words (e.g., "Based on your description, it sounds as though you are suffering with a depressive disorder")
Reflecting	Repeating key words to encourage the patient to keep speaking (e.g., He says: "I feel like a man on a desert island without water"; you say: "A man without water . . .")
Effective pause	To encourage the speaker to continue
Minimal encouragers	To encourage the speaker to continue (e.g., "uh huh," "OK," "I see," "that's interesting")
I-message	Expresses feelings to the individual in a nonthreatening manner (e.g., "I feel *frustrated* when you shout so angrily because *I am trying to help you . . . I'm on your side*"—an emotion, a behavior, and a reason are cited)
Open-ended questions	Questions that cannot be answered by a yes or no answer (e.g., "Tell me more about your relationship with your wife.")
Summarizing	"These seem to be the main concerns you have at this time . . ." "Based on what you've described, you feel this way about the current situation with your daughter . . ."

PSYCHOSOCIAL INTERVENTIONS
(FIGURE 4-1)

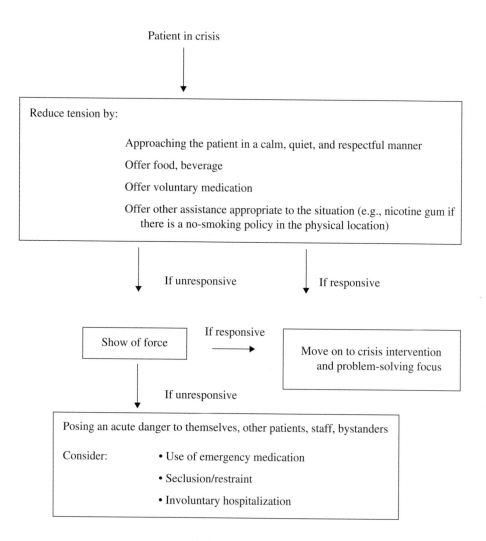

Figure 4-1   *Psychosocial Interventions Algorithm Summary.*

SOURCE: Allen et al. (2001). Reprinted with permission from McGraw-Hill.

RISK MANAGEMENT STRATEGIES

It is important to be thorough enough to accurately size up the factors that went into the making of the psychiatric emergency. The history of present illness (HPI) should include the biopsychosocial factors involved in the patient's current presentation (e.g., "Mr. Jones is a 35-year-old male with a lengthy history of schizophrenia, paranoid type. He presents today with a several-day history of decompensation due to increased alcohol abuse and poor psychotropic medication adherence. Mr. Jones has a family history of schizophrenia. His coping strategies typically involve drinking excessively, which he did this time after a fight with his girlfriend three days ago").

GAF is the Global Assessment of Functioning. It represents a continuum of mental health-illness. It is a 100-point scale that assesses an individual's level of psychological, social, and occupational functioning. It measures:

- Seriousness of the symptoms
- Seriousness of the impairment in school, work, and social function.

The GAF is a useful numerical way of categorizing the psychiatric emergency. It is probably most useful to record ratings over time (e.g., at admission and at discharge) to measure improvement as a function of treatment and the passage of time.

A biopsychosocial plan should also be documented. Recommendations for Mr. Jones might include:

Bio: Restart Zyprexa at 20 mg. Q hs.

Psych: Encourage sobriety and AA involvement to help develop healthier, sober coping strategies.

Social: Patient's sister is healthy and high-functioning; often she is the most reliable historian. Encourage him to talk with her. Also encourage him to attend day treatment regularly and request that the case manager monitor him more closely in the next 2 weeks.

Note how the patient responded to verbal interventions in the emergency situation. (e.g., "The patient was encouraged to vent his feelings and after about 10 minutes, he was able to calm down enough to discuss treatment options").

Often clinicians may want to give medication in order to feel something has been done. But this is not always wise or necessary. Give the patient, even the loud, angry patient, a chance to calm himself down with verbal intervention. Praise him for venting appropriately, express empathy for the pain he is feeling, and encourage the verbal expression of this painful feeling. Ask him what he needs to calm down. Certainly there are times clinicians hear expletives for a response. Try to hold ground and maintain a professional stance (e.g., "I'm here to help you in the situation. We can figure this out together. It's fine to talk out your feelings, but you know we can't have you get aggressive here with staff and other patients. We can sit down and talk this out and figure out what is best for you").

If this is a patient known to have hit staff—many charts have a label indicating this—a clinician should adjust his/her threshold of when it is time to abandon verbal interventions and move on to rapid control of the violent patient. This should be documented well (e.g., "Verbal interventions were attempted. The patient spit at this examiner and refused to follow directives to return to his room. Instead, he attempted to hit this examiner. Security was called; the patient was restrained for his own safety and protection as well as the safety and protection of others").

For the institution, ongoing staff training on techniques for crisis intervention is requisite.

BIBLIOGRAPHY

Allen M, et al. Treatment of Behavioral Emergencies. *Postgraduate Medicine* (May 2001): 1–88.

Diagnostic and Statistical Manual of Mental Disorders, 4th ed., Text Revision (DSM-IV-TR). Washington, DC: American Psychiatric Association, 2000.

Chapter 5

LEGAL PRINCIPLES

INTRODUCTION

It is essential for the clinician working in litigious times to understand the various medicolegal issues that impact the care of emergency psychiatric patients. The *Tarasoff* decision and duty to warn/protect has had a powerful influence on how mental health practitioners handle potentially violent patients. Understanding the features of civil commitment statutes, the definition of standard of care, and the documentation of solid, systematic clinical thinking is part of being an informed clinician.

The goals of this chapter include:

1. To define emergency
2. To review the major legal concepts relevant to mental health clinicians working in emergency situations, such as malpractice, informed consent, competence, confidentiality and privilege, seclusion/restraint and involuntary hospitalization/civil commitment, and patient dumping (COBRA/EMTALA)
3. To review risk management strategies for individual clinicians and institutions

EMERGENCY DEFINED

- A situation in which a patient, due to a mental disorder, poses an immediate risk to life and limb of self and others (Hillard, 1990)
- A set of circumstances in which a catastrophic outcome is thought to be imminent and the resources available to understand and deal with the situation are unavailable at the time and place of the occurrence (Allen, 1999)
- An unanticipated situation where the patient's behavior presents an immediate and serious danger to the safety of the patient, other patients, or staff (Resnick, 2000)
- May vary from state to state; the clinician should know the definition, if any, that exists in the state in which he/she practices

MAJOR LEGAL CONCEPTS (TABLE 5-1)

Professional liability claims against psychiatrists and other mental health professionals have increased markedly in recent years.

One out of every 12 psychiatrists can expect to be sued per year. The psychiatrist who works in the emergency setting and/or frequently treats suicidal/violent behavior patients also has a higher potential to be sued.

Clinicians in emergency settings are particularly at risk for such actions because of:

- High patient volume
- High level of acuity from patient dangerousness
- High level of acuity from patient medical complications
- Brief clinician-patient contacts

MALPRACTICE

Malpractice is a tort, a civil as opposed to a criminal wrong. In a malpractice suit, a plaintiff seeks to "become whole again" via financial compensation.

DUTY   In a psychiatric emergency setting, the clinician has a legal duty to evaluate within a reasonable period of time anyone who requests evaluation or who is legally brought in for evaluation. The clinician has the legal duty to provide whatever emergency treatment is indicated and to refer the patient appropriately. As will be discussed later in the chapter, the clinician also may have a legal duty to protect third parties who may be injured by the patient.

DERELICTION OR BREACH OF DUTY   A clinician is negligent if he or she fails to provide the standard of care that a reasonably prudent practitioner in the same specialty would provide under like or similar circumstances. In the past, the reference group has generally been the practitioners in the same locality. Currently, most jurisdictions favor a reference group consisting of practitioners nationwide. A practitioner need not do what a majority of colleagues would have done under similar circumstances, but the actions taken need to be endorsed by at least a respectable minority of practitioners to be considered to have met an acceptable standard of care. The APA's evidence-based practice guideline series help to establish a national uniformity to care.

The courts do not expect perfection and making an error in judgment is not the same as being negligent. If a patient commits suicide soon after leaving the emergency room, negligence is not assessed on the basis of what is known about the case after the fact, but on the basis of what was known or should have been known at the time the patient was seen. If an appropriate evaluation was conducted, and if reasonable conclusions were drawn from it and reasonable treatment was carried out, care is not likely to be found to have been negligent. Risk management strategies are discussed further at the conclusion of this chapter.

TABLE 5-1   THE 4 "DS" OF MALPRACTICE NEGLIGENCE

1. Duty—once a doctor-patient relationship is established, the doctor has a duty to treat the patient in accordance with the profession's standard of care
2. Dereliction or breach of duty
3. The dereliction or breach of duty is the direct cause of the damage
4. Damages result from the dereliction or breach of duty

DIRECT CAUSATION Medical thinking and legal thinking are two different types of thinking. For example, a psychiatrist might conceptualize a patient's suicide as multifactorial: it is the unfortunate result of an abusive childhood, a physical illness, unsupportive family, financial problems, and substance abuse.

A lawyer might view the proximate cause of the suicide as having been the physician's failure to foresee that the patient was incapable of complying with an outpatient referral. In general, the best test for whether a given act of negligence was the direct cause of damages is whether the damages were reasonably foreseeable on the basis of what the clinician knew or should have known.

DAMAGES Damages may be physical, financial, and/or emotional, but all damages are generally compensated financially. It is the charge of the judge and jury to reduce all damages to a specific dollar amount. Lawyers have access to data on the dollar amount of recent judgments in a particular locality and are able to state with some degree of accuracy what a given type of injury is worth in that locality (e.g., death by suicide of a father with a wife and a child under 5 years of age).

COMMON TYPES OF MALPRACTICE

Common types of psychiatric malpractice specific to the psychiatric emergency setting include:

- Failure to diagnosis suicide risk or risk of violence
- Failure to diagnose medical illness
- Inappropriate somatic treatment
- Inappropriate seclusion/restraint
- Failure to protect third parties from injury by dangerous patients

Since 1990, with the number of inpatient beds declining, malpractice claims have increased in outpatient settings. If a suicide occurs while a patient is on an inpatient unit, the clinician should expect there is a 1 in 2 likelihood of being sued (Slovenko, 1999).

The risk of a malpractice suit also increases with increased volume of patients seen. Psychiatrists who see more than 25 patients daily have a much higher risk of being sued. Also, a psychiatrist who takes on supervision responsibilities increases his/her likelihood of being sued the more supervisees he/she has under supervision (Stone, 1999).

INFORMED CONSENT (TABLE 5-2)

DEFINITION Medical and psychiatric treatment can only be undertaken with the patient's informed consent.

The concept of informed consent is rooted in two legal principles:

- The right of a patient to determine what will/will not be done to his/her body; the right of self-determination.
- The fiduciary nature of the doctor-patient relationship. Inherent in a fiduciary relationship is the responsibility of the physician to disclose honestly and in good faith all requisite facts involved in the treatment of the condition. This includes risks and benefits, alternatives and their consequences, and the consequences of no treatment. Such information is to promote autonomy and rational decision making on the part of the patient.

TABLE 5-2   **THE THREE MAIN ELEMENTS OF INFORMED CONSENT**

1. Competence—the patient is competent to give informed consent
2. Adequate information—the patient has been given adequate information to make informed consent possible
3. Voluntary—the consent is given voluntarily

COMPETENCE Competence is a legal term while capacity is a clinical term. However, for the purpose of this book, the authors will refer to competence.

A patient is presumed competent until proven otherwise. Competence is task-specific. This means that one may be competent in performing one task but not another (e.g., one may be competent to stand trial with the representation of a lawyer, but not competent to represent oneself pro se without a lawyer).

To be competent to make a specific clinical decision a patient should:

- Be aware of the clinical situation
- Have factual understanding of the issues involved
- Be able to manipulate the information rationally

Each state has a statute that defines general competence to handle affairs. Individuals who are incompetent can have a guardian appointed by the court. The guardian's judgment will substitute for that of the patient in clinical as well as in other situations. The guardian is charged by the court to act in the best interests of the incompetent individual.

Living wills and durable powers of attorney for health care decision making are now relatively common for medical care. However, the use of these legal tools in the psychiatric care arena has been less common.

When dealing with minors in the emergency setting, clarify quickly who is authorized to give treatment permission. Each state has a statutory definition of when an adolescent has reached the age of consent. Usually it is the parents who are the guardians of a minor unless guardianship has been transferred or unless the adolescent has been emancipated according to the laws of that state.

ADEQUATE INFORMATION This is information that a rational person would want to know when making a treatment decision and includes the following:

- What the medical and/or psychiatric condition is
- What the recommended treatment is
- What the risks and benefits of the recommended treatment are
- What the alternative treatments are
- What the risks and benefits of alternative treatments are
- What the risks and benefits of no treatment are

VOLUNTARY CONSENT Treatment decisions that are in any way coerced are not voluntary. For example, a patient told that "you can't leave the emergency room until you have had your medication" is not a patient who can give informed consent for the medication. Coercion and persuasion differ in that the former has the effect of undermining the patient's ability to reason while the latter aims to utilize the patient's reasoning ability to arrive at a desired result.

EXCEPTIONS TO INFORMED CONSENT (TABLE 5-3)

EMERGENCY. This was defined at the beginning of the chapter. In accordance with the earlier definition, this is a situation that requires immediate treatment to save the life or prevent imminent serious harm to patient and/or others. Two essential elements that define an emergency:

- A serious and imminent situation exists because of
- The patient's psychiatric condition

TABLE 5-3   **EXCEPTIONS TO INFORMED CONSENT**

1. Emergencies
2. Incompetence
3. Therapeutic privilege
4. Therapeutic waiver

INCOMPETENCE The patient lacks sufficient mental capacity to give informed consent and a substitute decision maker is either present or not.

THERAPEUTIC PRIVILEGE If a psychiatrist determines that a complete disclosure of possible risks might be injurious to the patient's health and welfare, he/she may choose not to disclose this information to the patient. This should never be done in order to avoid obtaining informed consent.

WAIVER If a patient competently, knowingly, and voluntarily waives his/her right to be informed, a physician need not disclose information (e.g., the patient says, "You're the Doc . . . just do whatever you think is best").

Remember that treatment without any consent or against the patient's wishes may constitute battery, an intentional tort. Treatment that is given without adequate consent could constitute an act of medical negligence.

CONFIDENTIALITY AND PRIVILEGE

DEFINITIONS

1. Confidentiality is the duty of the clinician not to disclose communications that took place in the doctor-patient relationship without written or verbal permission of the patient
2. Privilege is the legal right of the patient to forbid the doctor/clinic from disclosing information obtained in the context of the doctor-patient relationship in a legal proceeding

LIMITS TO CONFIDENTIALITY There are limits or exceptions to confidentiality that are mandated by law (Table 5-4).

Other exceptions to disclosure include:

• Communication within the team that is caring for the patient at a given agency. However, communication with the clinicians caring for the patient through other agencies is not acceptable unless the patient consents or unless another exception to confidentiality applies.
• When the patient is incompetent—in which case, the guardian's consent must be obtained. In the case of incompetent patients without guardians or family, the clinician must proceed and attempt to act in the best interests of the patient.
• When reporting is required by law (see Table 5-4). Some states also require a relative to be informed when a patient is involuntarily hospitalized.
• When the clinician is ordered to testify by a judge, the clinician must comply.
• When it is necessary to contact third parties to adequately evaluate a patient. This exception is particularly clear when a patient is brought in to be evaluated for involuntary hospitalization and it is impossible to make a reasonable decision about hospitalization without obtaining information from third parties.

TABLE 5-4 MANDATORY STATUTORY DISCLOSURE

1. Child abuse or neglect
2. Elder abuse or neglect
3. Duty to protect third parties (Tarasoff duty)
4. Past treasonous act
5. Intent to commit a future crime
6. HIV infection

SECLUSION/RESTRAINT (TABLES 5-5 AND 5-6)

The federal government (Centers for Medicare and Medicaid Services [CMS]), most states, and the Joint Commission on Accreditation of Healthcare Organizations (JCAHO) regulate the use of seclusion and restraint. Generally, restraints are to be used only when there is a risk of imminent harm to the patient and/or others and other less restrictive interventions have failed.

DEFINITIONS

1. **Seclusion:** The clinical definition of seclusion is the placing and retaining of a patient for the purpose of managing an emergency situation

   The statutory definition may specifically mandate a locked door; a subjective standard is the patient's own perception of having his movement limited

2. Restraint:
   - Personal—the application of physical force on a person's body without the use of any external device
   - Physical or mechanical—the application of physical force on a person's body utilizing a device attached or adjacent to his/her body

Chemical restraint is defined by federal law (H.R. 4365) as "the use of a drug or medication that is used as a restraint to control behavior or restrict the resident's freedom of movement that is not a standard treatment for the resident's medical or psychiatric condition." It is more accurate to characterize the use of antipsychotic medication as targeting and treating the psychosis (e.g., when a patient is agitated due to auditory hallucinations) (Cutler, 2000).

In the emergency situation it is sometimes necessary to seclude and/or restrain patients. Typically this occurs after sufficient efforts have been made to utilize less restrictive means of managing the patient (see Chapter 8, "The Potentially Violent Patient"). It is prudent to do so as swiftly, safely, and respectfully as possible.

In the PES or inpatient unit, the patient must be observed at minimum every 15 minutes.

TABLE 5-5 INDICATIONS FOR SECLUSION AND RESTRAINT

1. To prevent clear, imminent harm to the patient or others
2. To prevent significant disruption to treatment program or physical surroundings
3. To assist in treatment as part of ongoing behavior therapy
4. To decrease sensory overstimulation*
5. To comply with patient's voluntary reasonable request †

*Seclusion only
† First seclusion; then, if necessary, restraints.

TABLE 5-6 CONTRAINDICATIONS TO SECLUSION AND RESTRAINT

1. For extremely unstable medical and psychiatric conditions*
2. For patients with delirium or dementia who are unable to tolerate decreased stimulation*
3. For overtly suicidal patients*
4. For patients with severe drug reactions, those with overdoses, or those requiring close monitoring of drug dosages*
5. For punishment of the patient or convenience of the staff

*Unless close supervision and direct observation are provided.

There are times when a patient may require continuous observation or need to have a staff member in the seclusion room.

Document carefully what the clinical situation was and what efforts were tried before restraint was initiated. After the first hour of face-to-face assessment, the psychiatrist should see the patient at least every 3 hours. Document the patient's condition and why continued seclusion/restraint is necessary.

The use of seclusion and restraint may be indicated when other less restrictive interventions are ineffective or inappropriate. The goal is to prevent harm to the patient or other persons such as other patients, family, staff, or the public at large.

Use of seclusion and restraint is a matter of clinical judgment that should include a thorough understanding of the clinical needs of the patient and weighing the clinical risks and benefits of proceeding with the seclusion and/or restraint. Particular care should be taken in assessing the clinical need for seclusion and restraint in special populations such as children and adolescents, the elderly, and the developmentally disabled.

RESTRAINT REMOVAL   When the patient no longer poses an imminent threat to self or others and is no longer disruptive to the therapeutic setting, the removal of seclusion and restraint is permitted.

This is best accomplished in an incremental fashion. Each step should be carefully monitored for the patient's stability with increasing freedom of movement.

SECLUSION/RESTRAINT   CONTROVERSY   *This has been an area of increasing controversy over the last decade. In 1999, in response to deaths that occurred while patients were restrained, CMS (formerly the Health Care Financing Administration) initiated what some believed to be a stringent restraint policy. This policy has been criticized in particular for its failure to consider its economic impact on small, rural hospitals and residential treatment centers for children and adolescents.*[7]

This controversial 1-hour rule requires a licensed independent practitioner (LIP) or physician to see a patient face to face within 1 hour of ordering the seclusion and/or restraint. An LIP is an individual who is recognized by both state law and hospital policy as having the independent authority to order seclusion and restraints for patients; RNs, traditionally the authority on site, are not considered LIPs.

Critics of the CMS regulations also predict that more medications at higher doses will be given in an effort to prevent escalation to restraint. Supporters believe that such a policy will encourage safer, more creative, and less restrictive ways of dealing with such patients. The American Psychiatric Association Task Force on the Psychiatric Uses of Seclusion and Restraint (1985) and, more recently H.B. 4365, have established federal standards for seclusion and restraint. Two sets of standards are delineated: a more relaxed hospital-level standard and a more stringent residential treatment center–level standard (children/adolescents) (Cutler, 2000).

JCAHO will work to enforce CMS standards in hospitals receiving Medicaid and Medicare funding.

CIVIL COMMITMENT/INVOLUNTARY HOSPITALIZATION (TABLE 5-7)

For all intents and purposes, involuntary hospitalization and civil commitment are synonymous unless referring to outpatient commitment. Sometimes it becomes necessary for the outpatient clinician to initiate civil commitment on a patient. Typically state statutes define when this can be initiated and clinicians should know the law in their state.

If a physician fails to use the state commitment laws to involuntarily hospitalize a patient who clearly falls under those laws, the physician may have breached a legal duty. If a physician uses the state commitment laws to involuntarily hospitalize a patient who clearly does *not* fall under those laws, the physician may be guilty of having falsely imprisoned the patient. If force was necessary, the physician is probably exposed to battery charges also. In real clinical situations, it is often unclear whether a given patient meets the commitment laws. The best way to cope with

TABLE 5-7 TYPICAL SUBSTANTIVE AND MISCELLANEOUS CRITERIA FOR CIVIL COMMITMENT

Substantive criteria

1. Mentally ill
2. Dangerous to self or others
3. Unable to provide for basic needs

Miscellaneous criteria (in conjunction with one or more of the above criteria)

1. Gravely disabled (unable to care for self to the point of likely self-harm)
2. Refusing hospitalization
3. Patient is in need of hospitalization
4. Danger to property
5. Lacks capacity to make rational treatment decisions
6. Hospitalization represents the least restrictive alternative

---

this situation is to thoroughly understand the relevant laws and to try to apply them in good faith.

Liability for false imprisonment or battery is unlikely unless the physician acted maliciously or with reckless disregard for the truth or if false information was used to commit the patient (e.g., if a physician claims to have examined a patient whom he or she had never set eyes on). It is critical that the clinician fully document in the chart the rationale for whatever action was taken.

Since civil commitment and involuntary hospitalization are often necessary in the face of psychiatric emergencies, it is crucial that the clinician be familiar with the relevant state statutes.

The civil deprivation of a mentally ill person's freedom is premised on two legal doctrines:

• Police power: The state has the responsibility to safeguard its citizens; thus, the state has the right to detain a person who is mentally ill and a threat to others
• Parens patriae: The state has the responsibility to act on behalf of those citizens unable to care for themselves due to a mental illness

Toward the end of the twentieth century, emphasis on the dangerousness criteria in-creased. There has been much emphasis on the dangerousness criteria. This is likely due to stigma and misunderstandings about the relationship between mental illness and violence. The MacArthur Violence Risk Assessment Study helped clarify the relationship between mental illness and violence. Persons with mental illness do not commit most violent acts. However, there is a subset of patients who are more likely to be violent. Substance abuse is an important risk factor, significantly increasing the likelihood of violence perpetrated by the general population as well as the mentally ill (Steadman et al., 1998).

The presence of dangerousness without severe mental illness is not sufficient to involuntarily hospitalize a patient. Such persons are the responsibility of the police, not the psychiatrist.

Involuntary hospitalization is always a clinical intervention. Treat the patient with concern, respect, and fairness.

It is prudent to err on the side of safeguarding the lives of severely ill patients or endangered others by seeking hospitalization rather than giving precedence to preserving the patient's civil liberties. A patient who is likely to sign out against medical advice should be hospitalized involuntarily if the clinician believes the criteria are met for involuntary commitment.

PATIENT DUMPING

The Emergency Medical Treatment and Active Labor Act (EMTALA) delineates hospital transfer guidelines. EMTALA is part of the Consolidated Omnibus Budget Reconciliation Act (COBRA) originally passed by Congress in 1985. EMTALA was intended to remove economic considerations from medical decision making in the emergency department. Hospital and physicians are required to stabilize patients prior to transfer to another institution. This includes psychiatric patients who may, for example, be experiencing substance withdrawal or an acute psychotic episode. Increased scrutiny of hospitals and physicians and enforcement of EMTALA by CMS and private citizens is likely in the future.

RISK MANAGEMENT STRATEGIES

FOR THE INDIVIDUAL CLINICIAN

- Do what is clinically appropriate; a good-faith attempt to care for the patient in a clinically appropriate way is generally the best defense
- Know the state statutes and any hallmark common-law court verdicts relevant to mental health
- Remember that imminent risk to life and limb usually overrides other considerations such as confidentiality, informed consent, or false imprisonment
- Try, as much as possible, to get informed consent from the patient and the family, even if a patient is to be hospitalized involuntarily
- Talk with the patient and family enough that they do not leave angry; effective communication can prevent lawsuits in certain situations
- Document evaluation, clinical decision making, and treatment in the medical record

  Specifically:
  - Make sure that the assessment and plans are supported by the subjective and objective data recorded

- Document contact with third parties
- Include pertinent negatives (e.g., patient has made no previous suicide attempts)
- Explain rationale for controversial decisions (e.g., "Although this patient poses some long-term risk of suicide, hospitalization is not indicated since his long-term treatment plan calls for maximum effort at outpatient problem resolution and since the acute risk of suicide is past, as evidenced by . . .")
- Make sure that any negative countertransference feelings about the patient are not reflected in the chart
- Seek consultation or independent assessment of difficult patients
- Routinely request and examine old records and get, with the patient's consent, information from other clinicians treating the patient
- Accept the probability of eventually being sued; make sure that you have legal consultation available and adequate professional liability insurance

FOR THE INSTITUTION

- Provide adequate staffing
- Provide as safe an environment as reasonably possible
- Provide risk management and legal backup
- Provide patient relations and ombudsman service
- Provide adequate medical and surgical backup
- Have written, and easily followed, policies and procedures and documentation protocols
- Have periodic quality-assurance audits
- Screen patients quickly after they arrive to determine which need immediate attention and which can wait
- Make consultation available, at least by phone
- Have explicit understandings with referral agencies, disposition sites, and managed-care systems
- Have orientation meetings with appropriate institutional resources to clarify any potential problems, conflicts, etc.

- Have sound credentialing policies to make sure you have a competent clinical staff

Specifically in regard to seclusion and restraint:

- Staff should be thoroughly trained in the use of alternative interventions that may reduce the need for seclusion and restraint
- Staff should be thoroughly trained in the safe and effective techniques for implementing seclusion and restraint
- Restraint should be applied only with sufficient numbers of staff present to help ensure a safe and effective implementation of seclusion and restraint
- Hospitals should engage in a continuous quality improvement process that seeks to minimize the use of seclusion and restraint consistent with good standards of clinical practice and the needs of individual patients
- Death or serious injury resulting from interventions involving seclusion and restraint must be reviewed internally; in addition to internal review, external review by or subject to an accrediting organization may also be required, with appropriate legal and confidentiality protections

BIBLIOGRAPHY

Allen MH. Level I Psychiatric Emergency Services: The Tools of the Crisis Sector. *Psychiatric Clinics of North America* 22(4) (1999): 714.

American Psychiatric Association. *The Psychiatric Uses of Seclusion and Restraint* (Task Report no 22). Washington, DC: American Psychiatric Press, 1985; amended 1992.

COBRA/EMTALA Online Federal Regulations 489.24 (1985).

Cutler JB. *APA Seclusion and Restraint Legislative Update.* http://www.psych.org.

Hillard JR, ed. *Manual of Clinical Emergency Psychiatry.* Washington, DC: American Psychiatric Press, 1990.

Resnick PJ. *American Academy of Psychiatry and Law Review Course Syllabus.* Vancouver: 2000.

Slovenko R. Malpractice in Psychotherapy: An Overview. *Psychiatric Clinics of North America* 22(2) (1999): 1–15.

Steadman H, Mulvey E, Monahan J, Robbins P, Appelbaum P, Grisso T, Roth L, Silver E. Violence by People Discharged from Acute Psychiatric Inpatient Facilities and by Others in the Same Neighborhoods. *Archives of General Psychiatry* 55 (1998): 1–9.

Stone AA. Managed Care, Liability, and ERISA. *Psychiatric Clinics of North America* 22(2) (1999): 17–29.

Chapter 6

PSYCHIATRIC ETHICS

INTRODUCTION

Common sense is important in clinical decision making, but common sense alone is not enough. A clinician must have an understanding of ethics concepts and be able to systematically apply them to often-complex psychiatric decisions. In order to optimize both ethical and clinical reasoning, clinicians should make every effort to suspend moral judgments.

The goals of this chapter include:

1. Define key concepts of psychiatric ethics including ethics, morals, principles, and rights
2. Outline the classical and alternative ethical frameworks applied to clinical decision making; these include:

- Utilitarian
- Deontological (Kantian)
- Paternalism
- Virtue theory
- Ethics of care
- Casuistry

3. Outline a framework of moral principles designed to assist the ethically responsible clinician in identifying and reflecting on moral problems
4. Recommend approaches to common emergency psychiatry ethical dilemmas
5. Brief review of AMA Principles of Medical Ethics with Annotations Especially Applicable to Psychiatry
6. Risk management strategies

DEFINITIONS

1. **Ethics:** The body of moral principles or values governing a particular culture or group; a complex of moral precepts held or rules of conduct followed by an individual; high standards of honest and honorable dealing and of methods used, especially in the professions or in business.

   Do not confuse ethics with morals; ethics has to do with the way one thinks about and discusses moral problems.
2. **Morals:** Generally accepted customs of conduct and right living in a society and the individual's practice in relation to these.
3. **Principles:** Accepted or professed rules of action or conduct; fundamental doctrines claiming that acts have validity without specific regard to their consequences; a guiding sense of the requirements and obligations of right conduct; a general and fundamental truth that may be used in deciding conduct or choice
4. **Rights:** Acknowledged interests within a moral or a legal system that (usually) impose an obligation on others
5. **Ethical reasoning:** A rational process of choosing the most morally desirable course of action
6. **Ethical dilemma:** A conflict between competing values or principles of conduct, e.g., preserving a patient's liberty vs. detaining a patient involuntarily or preserving confidentiality vs. violating confidentiality to fulfill a Tarasoff duty to protect third parties

CLASSICAL ETHICAL THEORIES

1. Utilitarian
   - The object of morality is to promote human welfare by minimizing harms and maximizing benefits
   - The emphasis is on consequences of acts with the choices leading to the greatest possible welfare of all concerned
2. Deontological or Kantian
   - Acts are morally praiseworthy only if the person's motive for acting is to perform a true duty. For example, a psychiatric resident stays up all night with an unstable manic patient. If he did so to gain the respect of his attending physician or to avoid litigation, he deserves no moral praise. If he did so out of a pure sense of duty to the patient, his actions are morally praiseworthy.
   - The emphasis is on treating others as ends in and of themselves, not as the means to the clinician's selfish ends

ALTERNATIVES TO CLASSICAL THEORIES

1. Virtue theory
   - The cultivation of virtuous traits of character is the central feature of the moral life; thus, the virtuous character will make sound ethical decisions.
2. The ethics of care
   - The focus is on features of close personal relationships such as sympathy, fidelity, love, and friendship applied to clinician-patient relationships.
3. Casuistry
   - This is analogous to the case law concept: current decision making is based on judgments reached in prior cases.

A FRAMEWORK OF MORAL PRINCIPLES

The following are five principles that can aid the clinician in identifying and reflecting on moral problems.

1. Respect for autonomy (respecting the decision-making capacities of autonomous persons)
2. Nonmaleficence (avoiding the causation of harm)
3. Beneficence (providing benefits and balancing benefits against risks)
4. Justice (fairness in the distribution of benefits and risks)
5. Fidelity (responsibility to the patient is paramount)

PATERNALISM

1. The clinician acts as a parent; she treats the patient as a child who cannot determine his own good
2. Behavior is paternalistic when it satisfies four criteria:
   * It is carried out with the intent of benefiting the patient.
   * It involves the violation of a moral rule with respect to the patient. Violating a moral rule involves acting toward someone in a way that either directly inflicts a harm (e.g., death, pain, disability, loss of freedom/pleasure), or increased likelihood that the person will suffer one or more harms.
   * It is carried out without the consent of the patient.
   * The patient is at least partially competent or is expected to become at least partially competent in the future.
3. Paternalistic behavior is justified if:
   * The harms the treatment will avoid or ameliorate must be very great.
   * The harms imposed by the treatment are less by comparison.
   * The patient's desire not to be treated is seriously irrational.
   * Rational persons would advocate always allowing forced treatment in cases having the same morally relevant characteristics described by the above three criteria.

AMA PRINCIPLES OF MEDICAL ETHICS WITH ANNOTATIONS ESPECIALLY APPLICABLE TO PSYCHIATRY

This is a set of fairly straightforward, practical principles (e.g., "A physician shall be dedicated to providing competent medical service with compassion and respect for human dignity"). The full text can be found on the Web site of the APA and clinicians are urged to familiarize themselves with this document. It is important to remember, however, that "immutable ethical rules are simply not available." Clinicians are responsible for making ethical decisions in specific cases.

ETHICAL WORKUP (TABLE 6-1)

Document systematically

1. Describe relevant biological, psychological, and social facts
2. Describe the ethical and legal perspective
3. Note the principal value conflicts
4. Note the possible courses of action
5. Choose and defend course of action

ETHICS AND SUICIDAL BEHAVIOR

This is a common emergency psychiatry situation. Here the dilemma is between limiting autonomy (involuntarily hospitalizing a patient) vs. preserving autonomy (and placing the patient in a potentially lethal situation). For patients determined to be at a high risk of suicide, the authors advocate limiting autonomy in order to ultimately preserve autonomy. In other words, such patients should be involuntarily hospitalized to help them regain the freedom lost temporarily to:

1. Psychiatric disorder
2. Overwhelming stress
3. Difficult interpersonal relationships

ETHICS AND VIOLENT BEHAVIOR

This is another common emergency psychiatry situation. Here the dilemma is preserving patient confidentiality and safeguarding the privacy that is so essential to honest, open, authentic communication between the therapist and the patient vs. the clinician's Tarasoff duty to protect third parties from being harmed by their dangerous patients. Preserving life is the highest moral value and trumps other concerns.

ETHICS AND INFORMED CONSENT

In an emergency situation it is unnecessary to obtain informed consent. However, it is preferable to inform the patient of the various components of informed consent when he is able to understand.

ETHICS AND INVOLUNTARY COMMITMENT

Emergency situations in psychiatry often lead to involuntary detainment. If the patient is at risk of harm to self/others, is unable to care for his/her basic needs, or would benefit from hospitalization, this fulfills the legal criteria necessary to hospitalize. Paternalistic thinking (reviewed above in "Paternalism") often guides the clinician's decision-making process in the case of involuntary detainment.

TABLE 6-1   THREE TESTS TO USE IN DETERMINING THE RIGHT COURSE OF ACTION

1. Impartiality: *Would you be willing to have this action performed if you were in the patient's place?*
2. Universalizability: *Are you willing to have this action performed in all relevantly similar circumstances?*
3. Interpersonal justifiability: *Are you able to provide good reasons to justify your actions to others?*

ETHICS AND RATIONING HEALTH CARE: ETHICS AND ECONOMIC OR FINANCIAL FACTORS

As the number of inpatient beds continues to decline and community resources remain scarce, it is likely that admissions to emergency psychiatry facilities will continue to increase. In 1970 there were 524,878 inpatient beds in the United States; by 1998, the number dropped by about 50% to 261,903.

It is common to have multiple patients in a PES "waiting for a bed to open up." It is a common refrain to hear that "beds are tight in the city" and those that are available go quickly. Who should get the bed? An insured patient vs. an uninsured patient? Some inpatient facilities have agreements to hospitalize a certain number of indigent patients; the preference is to take on insured patients. Typically, it is first come, first serve. Those patients who have been deemed to need inpatient care will be assigned a bed in the order in which they presented to the emergency department.

ETHICS AND MANAGED CARE

Managed care companies, in which a physician is often financially rewarded for limiting care, dominate the health care system at this time. In emergency situations, it is prudent that the physician remember that his/her fiduciary duty is to the patient and take care to make clinical decisions based on the best interest of the patient.

ETHICS OF CONFIDENTIALITY AND DOUBLE AGENTRY

Double agentry involves the psychiatrist in conflicting roles:

1. Obligation to the patient
2. Obligation to an innocent third party
3. Obligation to the institution for which the psychiatrist is employed
3. Obligations to society at large

RISK MANAGEMENT

Clinicians should:

- Be familiar with APA guidelines of ethical conduct.
- Be in the habit of utilizing a systematic way of thinking through ethical issues involved in clinical decision making.
- Remember that legal does not equal moral. A clinician should arrive at his own conclusions/"code" of what is right.
- Constantly update knowledge; self-scrutinize and raise their own moral consciousness.
- Suspend common moral judgments in emergency settings in order to optimize both clinical and ethical reasoning. Repeaters in the PES are frustrating for staff and it is tempting to become negative and judgmental with such patients. Ours is not to judge. Ours is to form clinical judgments based on a bio/psycho/social model that will guide management.
- Remember to wisely use one's power to diagnose, hospitalize, and/or force treatment, keeping the patient's best interest always in the forefront.

BIBLIOGRAPHY

Bloch S, et al. *Psychiatric Ethics*, 3rd ed. Oxford: Oxford University Press, 1999.

The Principles of Medical Ethics with Annotations Especially Applicable to Psychiatry. Washington, DC: American Psychiatric Association, 1995.

PART II

Clinical Challenges in Emergency Psychiatry

Chapter 7

THE POTENTIALLY SUICIDAL PATIENT

INTRODUCTION

Approximately 30,000 Americans commit suicide every year. Many saw either a primary care physician or a mental health professional within a year and, in some cases, within a month of committing suicide.

Major mental disorders are associated with an increased risk of suicide. Major depression may result in suicide completion in 15% of afflicted patients. Ten to fifteen percent of patients with bipolar disorder and 10% of schizophrenic patients are estimated to complete suicide. Substance use disorders compound the risk of suicide for all of these disorders; 15% of patients with substance use disorders complete suicide.

The goals of this chapter include:

1. Review definitions of suicide and parasuicidal behavior
2. Review risk factors for suicidality
3. Review interview strategies
4. Review risk assessment and suicide risk factors checklist
5. Review management of the suicidal patient in an emergency setting
6. Review age/gender/cultural considerations

DEFINITIONS

1. Suicide is the intentional ending of one's own life
2. Parasuicidal behaviors are suicidal gestures or behaviors designed to bring concern and attention to oneself rather than the intention to die

RISK FACTORS (TABLE 7-1)

TABLE 7-1 **SUICIDE RISK FACTORS**

Age—adolescent and elderly
Male
Single, widowed
Poor physical health
Mental illness, such as mood disorder, schizophrenia, substance abuse
Caucasian
Feelings of hopelessness, helplessness
Isolation
Unemployment or stressful work situation
Poor financial situation
Previous suicide attempt
Family history of completed or attempted suicide

INTERVIEWING THE POTENTIALLY SUICIDAL PATIENT

Suicidal patients are comprised of:

- Those referred after a suicide attempt
- Those presenting with suicidal thoughts or plans
- Those presenting with other psychiatric or substance use disorders

For those referred after a suicide attempt, for example from the emergency department (ED), it is important to determine the events that led to the suicide attempt. A frequent presentation to the psychiatric emergency service (PES) setting is the individual who is being referred from an ED post overdose and stomach decontamination procedures. The ED doctor calls up and reports the information and asks for a referral to the PES setting if one exists or, in a consultative model, asks for psychiatric consultation to the ED.

Determine the relationship between lethality and rescue. Was this a high-lethality/low-rescue situation? For example, the individual checked into a hotel, wrote a note, and ingested a bottle of pills. Or was this an impulsive low-lethality/high-rescue situation? For example, after a fight with her boyfriend, a girl ran into the bathroom and swallowed a bottle of aspirin while he pounded on the bathroom door. While both may say "overdose" on the ED note, they are very different in terms of the lethality/rescue ratio.

Questions/issues to explore during an interview may include:

- What are the precipitating stressors? For example, relationship breakup, a recent death or loss? A medical or physical health change? Explore when and why the patient began to feel suicidal and what plans may have taken shape in his/her mind.
- Ask why now? Ask how the patient has handled situations like this in the past. For example, when he/she has felt so bad he/she wanted to die, how did he/she cope with those feelings?
- Has the individual attempted suicide before?
- What is the lethality of past attempts?

- If the individual attempted suicide with true intent, how does he/she feel about waking up alive? Often patients will feel ashamed and embarrassed, but glad to be alive. They may be eager to go home and get on with their lives. But there are those who wake up disappointed to be alive.
- Does the individual wish he/she had succeeded?
- Would he/she try it again?
- How many times has she tried to commit suicide?
- By what means? What means are available to her?
- Family history of suicide?

For those patients presenting with complaints of other mental disorders, it is important to ask about suicidal ideation/intent/plans in order to be thorough and complete in the exam.

SUICIDE RISK ASSESSMENT

THE DIFFICULTY OF RISK ASSESSMENT

A number of suicide risk assessment tools have been devised (e.g., self-report instruments such as the Beck Suicide Ideation Inventory). We know that postmortem brains of suicide victims have low serotonin 5-HT metabolites, adding further support for the SSRI treatment of depression. Still, many of the tools devised have an estimated 30% false-positive meaning and still other studies have shown us that there is no way to predict suicide, that the infrequency of an event such as suicide makes it all the more difficult to predict.

As yet, we do not have a biological marker in vivo that can predict suicide. Suicide probably involves too complex an interplay of factors—historical, biological, interpersonal, cultural, and religious, for example—to ever be able to identify a biological marker that could predict for its occurrence.

Having said all the above, mental health clinicians are expected to be able to predict violence in others and risk of violence to oneself.

A PARADIGM SHIFT

There has been a paradigm shift from predicting suicide as a yes-or-no, one-time prediction to assessing risk for suicide (e.g., low, moderate, high, imminent).

A SUICIDE RISK CHECKLIST

A suicide risk assessment utilizing a checklist may be helpful in guiding a systematic evaluation of these individuals (Table 7-2). The checklist in Table 7-2 conceptualizes individual factors as inhibiting or facilitating suicide and helps to guide the clinician at arriving at a level of risk for the unique patient at hand. The intent is to improve upon unaided clinical evaluations and to increase the safety of patients.

A word of caution about checklists. They inform professional judgment; they are not a substitute. One check on the checklist could mean high or imminent risk or could mean low risk. If other factors unique to this patient are noted, they should be considered.

TABLE 7-2 SUICIDE RISK CHECKLIST

Risk Factor	Facilitating Suicide	Inhibiting Suicide
Demographic		
Age	_____	_____
Sex	_____	_____
Marital status	_____	_____
Race	_____	_____
Individual		
Unique, characteristic patient factors	_____	_____
Clinical		
Current attempt (lethality/rescue ratio)	_____	_____
Panic attacks	_____	_____
Psychic anxiety	_____	_____
Loss of pleasure and interest	_____	_____
Substance abuse	_____	_____
Depressive turmoil	_____	_____
Diminished concentration	_____	_____
Global insomnia	_____	_____
Suicide plan	_____	_____
Suicide ideation	_____	_____
Suicide intent	_____	_____
Hopelessness	_____	_____
Prior attempts (lethality/rescue ratio)	_____	_____
Axis I diagnosis	_____	_____
Axis II diagnosis	_____	_____
Recent discharge from the hospital (3 months)	_____	_____
Impulsivity	_____	_____
Physical illness	_____	_____
Family history of suicide	_____	_____
Mental competency	_____	_____
Recent humiliation	_____	_____
Situational	_____	_____
Living circumstances	_____	_____
Employment status	_____	_____
Financial status	_____	_____
Availability of lethal means (e.g., guns)	_____	_____
Managed-care setting	_____	_____
Overall risk rating	_____	_____

SOURCE: Adapted from Simon R. *Concise Guide to Psychiatry and Law for Clinicians.* Arlington, VA: American Psychiatric Press, 1997 (hereafter Simon 1997).

DOCUMENTATION OF SUICIDE RISK ASSESSMENT AND RISK REDUCTION PLAN (TABLE 7-3)

In the psychiatric emergency setting a clinician will likely complete one risk assessment that will determine intervention, i.e., inpatient vs. outpatient plan. If the patient is admitted, the risk assessment would be done serially on the inpatient unit, particularly after each shift in terms of increased freedom of movement, post change in privilege level in the hospital, after home visits, upon discharge, at return appointments. See Table 7-3 for guidelines on documentation.

A WORD ON "NO-SUICIDE CONTRACTS"

Most clinicians are well aware by now that "no-suicide contracts" have no legal value in and of themselves. The most protective action from a patient safety and professional liability viewpoint is to complete and document a suicide risk assessment as outlined. Emphasizing therapeutic rapport and cooperation between the patient and clinician is a good idea. A no-suicide contract may then best be seen as adjunctive to a suicide risk assessment and risk reduction plan.

THE SOCIOECONOMICALLY DEPRIVED PATIENT

A disturbing trend in the urban PES is the homeless and possibly mentally ill socioeconomically deprived patient, who comes in announcing suicidal intentions in order to be hospitalized. Such patients are undoubtedly in dire straits. They are homeless, often using drugs, involved in crime, impoverished, poorly educated with no appreciable job skills, and have a whole host of ills. To compound matters, they are often their own worst enemies, having burned bridges with treatment providers by not showing up or exploiting services. Such patients are desperate certainly and they present seeking hospitalization to get warm (East Coast winters are bitterly cold) and in some ways it is a sensible way of solving a problem in their world of limited resources.

A clinician may ask herself: Do I admit a patient that I think is malingering? Do I spend time helping him figure out other more appropriate options and essentially ignore the suicide complaints by seeing them for what they are (i.e., need for basic services such as shelter, warmth, food, health care, with the occasional attempt to avoid police or others in the neighborhood)?

TABLE 7-3 **FEATURES OF THE CLINICIAN'S NOTE REGARDING RISK FACTORS**

The risk factors for this unique and individual patient
The protective factors for this unique and individual patient
Your estimate of level of risk based on your clinical interview and use of checklist
Your risk reduction plan for this individual

PRESCRIBING ANTIDEPRESSANT MEDICATIONS FROM THE PSYCHIATRIC EMERGENCY DEPARTMENT

Once a thorough evaluation is conducted, the clinician forms a risk management plan. A patient deemed at high or imminent risk of suicide should be placed on suicide precautions while an inpatient hospitalization is arranged.

If the patient is not an imminent risk of suicide, she can be referred to outpatient care.

Another option is to initiate antidepressant medication from the PES setting.

This is somewhat controversial since the clinician is seeing this individual under less-than-ideal circumstances (i.e., often without benefit of prior treatment records or access to other treatment providers). The clinical snapshot is thus brief. The authors do think it is appropriate under some circumstances to initiate antidepressant medications from the psychiatric emergency service. We caution that clinicians prescribe limited amounts of antidepressant medications. Ideally, an appointment with a psychiatrist within a week of the psychiatric emergency is preferred, thus allowing that community treatment provider to conduct a more thorough psychiatric evaluation to inform their choice of the best psychotropic medication(s). However, the authors recognize the reality of long waits for such appointments, combined with the typical latency period before antidepressant medications take effect and the risks of untreated depression. We recommend that clinicians weigh the risks with the benefits of prescribing antidepressant medications and act humanely.

The clinician may call the outpatient mental health clinic to speak with the medical director about concerns and perceived need that the patient be seen within a week instead of 2 months. But often the resources are simply not in place and the patient will have to wait. Referral to the patient's primary care physician may also be an option. Depending on the PES clinician's own comfort level and availability, he/she may opt to begin treatment on antide-pressants from the emergency room, give no more than 1 week's supply, and have the patient return until the outpatient linkage is made. This is controversial because of liability concerns in extending the role and responsibility for the patient beyond the emergency clinician role. Also, in the authors' experience, the PES is often too busy to accommodate these outpatient appointments. Still, if a patient is willing to wait, it may be a reasonable solution to the difficulty of getting prompt outpatient appointments.

AGE/GENDER/CULTURAL CONSIDERATIONS

Adolescent and elderly populations continue to grow in terms of risk of suicide. Females make 3–4 times the attempts that males do, and males have an increased rate of completion compared to females. The clinician should consider the subculture of the individual patient, the values of that subculture, and the degree of the cultural influences on the individual patient. For example, we know that the Catholic religion specifically prohibits the taking of one's own life. Asking the individual about his religious beliefs may help to shed light on his risk of suicide.

Most religions prohibit suicide. How does the individual patient fit into this? Do not presume that social embeddedness, being part of one's community and church, is a protective factor for suicide. It has been presumed that African-American women have the highest social embeddedness, but a recent study showed that might not be true. Do not presume based on cultural stereotypes that an individual patient is involved in such activities. Ask.

Widowed men, particularly young widowed males, are at greater risk of suicide. Ask about the status and healthiness of the marriage or relationship. Some literature suggests that homosexuality may also increase suicide risk; specifically, gay teens or teens with sexual identity issues may be at a higher risk for suicide.

BIBLIOGRAPHY

American Psychiatric Association. *Practice Guidelines for the Treatment of Patients with Suicidal Behaviors.* http://www.psych.org.

Baldessarini RJ, Jamison KR. Effects of Medical Interventions on Suicidal Behavior: Summary and Conclusions. *Journal of Clinical Psychiatry* 60(Suppl. 2) (1999): 117–22.

Beautrais AL. Gender Issues in Youth Suicidal Behaviour. *Emergency Medicine* 14(1) (March 2002): 35–42. Review.

Caine ED, Conwell Y. Suicide in the Elderly. *International Journal of Clinical Psychopharmacology* 16(Suppl. 2) (March 2001): S25–30. Review.

Cochrane-Brink KA, Lofchy JS, Sakinofsky I. Clinical Rating Scales in Suicide Risk Assessment. *General Hospital Psychiatry* 22(6) (November–December 2000): 445–51.

Conwell Y. Management of Suicidal Behavior in the Elderly. *Psychiatric Clinics of North America* 20(3) (September 1997): 667–83. Review.

Frierson RL, Melikian M, Wadman PC. Principles of Suicide Risk Assessment: How to Interview Depressed Patients and Tailor Treatment. *Postgraduate Medicine* 112(3) (September 2002): 65–66, 69–71.

Hawton K, Harriss L, Hodder K, Simkin S, Gunnell D. The Influence of the Economic and Social Environment on Deliberate Self-harm and Suicide: An Ecological and Person-based Study. *Psychological Medicine* 31(5) (July 2001): 827–36.

Hirschfeld RM. When to Hospitalize Patients at Risk for Suicide. *Annals of New York Academy of Science* 932 (April 2001): 188–96; discussion 196–99.

Kelly TM, Cornelius JR, Lynch KG. Psychiatric and Substance Use Disorders as Risk Factors for Attempted Suicide among Adolescents: A Case Control Study. *Suicide and Life-Threatening Behavior* 32(3) (Fall 2002): 301–12.

Lester D. Quality of Life for Children and Suicide Rates. *Psychological Report* 89(3) (December 2001): 616.

Luoma JB, Martin CE, Pearson JL. Contact with Mental Health and Primary Care Providers before Suicide: A Review of the Evidence. *American Journal of Psychiatry* 159(6) (June 2002): 909–16. Review.

Luoma JB, Pearson JL. Suicide and Marital Status in the United States, 1991–1996: Is Widowhood a Risk Factor? *American Journal of Public Health* 92(9) (September 2002): 1518–22.

Maris RW. Suicide. *Lancet* 360(9329) (July 27, 2002): 319–26.

Neeleman J. Beyond Risk Theory: Suicidal Behavior in Its Social and Epidemiological Context. *Crisis* 23(3) (2002): 114–20.

Neeleman J, Wessely S, Lewis G. Suicide Acceptability in African- and White Americans: The Role of Religion. *Journal of Nervous Mental Disorders* 186(1) (January 1998): 12–16.

Rutter PA, Soucar E. Youth Suicide Risk and Sexual Orientation. *Adolescence* 37(146) (Summer 2002): 289–99.

Shiang J. Does Culture Make a Difference? Racial/Ethnic Patterns of Completed Suicide in San Francisco, CA 1987–1996 and Clinical Applications. *Suicide and Life-Threatening Behavior* 28(4) (Winter 1998): 338–54.

Simon RI. Suicide Risk Assessment: What Is the Standard of Care? *Journal of the American Academy of Psychiatry and Law* 30(3) (2002): 340–44.

Snowden LR. Social Embeddedness and Psychological Well-being among African Americans and Whites. *American Journal of Community Psychology* 29(4) (August 2001): 519–36.

Chapter 8

THE POTENTIALLY VIOLENT PATIENT

INTRODUCTION

A critical role of the emergency clinician is to decide who is at risk for violent behavior. And once that is decided, what is the best course of action? Risk assessment is crucial and must be systematic, despite the external and internal pressures to move quickly in the psychiatric emergency setting.

Substance use and substance-induced disorders abound in the psychiatric emergency setting and clinicians need to be aware that these patients are at particularly high risk (above all other major psychiatric diagnoses) for violence. The MacArthur Violence Risk Assessment Study answered many questions regarding the relationship between mental illness and violence.

Findings of the MacArthur Violence Risk Assessment include the following:

- There is a weak relationship between mental illness and violence; most mentally ill people are generally not violent
- If violent conduct occurs, it is greater only during acute psychiatric symptoms
- Victims of the mentally ill are rarely strangers; they are more typically family members or friends
- Substance abuse is a much greater risk fac-

tor for violence than mental illness; there is no significant difference between the prevalence of violence by non-substance-abusing patients without symptoms of substance abuse and the prevalence of violence by others living in the same neighborhoods who were also non-substance abusers

The goals of this chapter include:

1. Define violence and violent behaviors
2. Review developmental factors associated with adult violence
3. Review diagnoses/symptoms that are commonly associated with violent behavior
4. Review working relationships with police and security personnel
5. Review clinician demeanor and interview strategies with potentially violent patients (Stay Cool mnemonic)
6. Review the paradigm shift from predicting dangerousness to assessing violence risk
7. Review the key features of violence risk assessment in a psychiatric emergency situation including culture/age/gender factors as they relate to violence
8. Review assessment and management of the potentially violent patient in the emergency situation to protect the patient and others (for psychotropic medication interventions see Chapter 3)

9. Review the Tarasoff duty to warn/protect third parties from dangerous patients
10. Risk management strategies

DEFINITIONS

Affective aggression is the result of external and internal threatening stimuli that evoke an intense and patterned activation of the autonomic nervous system, accompanied by threatening vocalizations and attacking or defending postures. This is characteristic of violence seen in psychiatric emergencies.

Foreshadowing behaviors include:

- Clenching of fists, jaw
- Pacing
- Sitting on the edge of the chair and clutching the armrest of the chair
- Slamming doors, banging their fists on a wall
- Hitting the palms of their hands with their fists
- Jumpy and easy to startle

Predatory aggression is planned, purposeful, and goal-directed. Unlike affective aggression, it is not reactive and requires emotional detachment. This is the hallmark of the psychopathic character. It is exceedingly dangerous because there are no behaviors that foreshadow it. It is atypical in psychiatric emergencies.

Behavior that is fear-inducing to the average person may be counted as violence. Physical and psychological manifestations of violence may include: kicking, screaming, slapping, punching, hitting, biting, spitting, threatening, intrusion into psychic space, hair pulling, brandishing an object as a weapon toward innocent others, and stalking; all may cause fear for those involved.

Hughes (1996) estimates that:

- 17% of psychiatric emergency service (PES) patients are suicidal
- 17% are homicidal
- 5% are both

DEVELOPMENTAL FACTORS ASSOCIATED WITH ADULT VIOLENCE

Childhood factors correlated with later violence include:

- Abuse by parents
- Truancy, school failures, lower IQ
- Delinquency as an adolescent
- Arrest for prior assault
- Childhood hyperactivity or serious inattention
- First psychiatric hospitalization by age 18
- Fire setting and animal cruelty
- History of being a childhood bully

DIAGNOSES/SYMPTOMS COMMONLY ASSOCIATED WITH VIOLENT BEHAVIOR

It is imperative in the PES setting to first consider whether a general medical condition(s) is present and, if so, whether such a condition is contributory or merely incidental to the patient's presentation (Table 8-1). See Chapter 1, "Emergency Medicine Approach to Psychiatric Illness."

Substance use disorders top the list of diagnoses associated with violence. Substance intoxication impairs judgment and social and occupational functioning. Intoxication with substances such as phencyclidine, cocaine, or amphetamine may lead to interpersonal sensi-tivity; cocaine and amphetamine intoxication syndromes are associated with anxiety, anger, and tension. Belligerence, assaultiveness, and impulsiveness are among the criteria for phen-cyclidine intoxication. Alcohol intoxication is associated with inappropriate sexual or aggressive behavior and impaired judgment.

Axis II personality disorders associated with violence include paranoid personality disorder and cluster B personality disorders such as antisocial personality disorder, narcissistic personality disorder, and borderline personality disorder (Table 8-2).

Table 8-3 lists specific psychotic symptoms that may be associated with increased risk of violence.

TABLE 8-1 **SCHIZOPHRENIA, PARTICULARLY PARANOID SCHIZOPHRENIA, PATIENTS MAY BE AT RISK, ESPECIALLY IN THE ACTIVE PHASES OF THEIR ILLNESS, TO COMMIT VIOLENT ACTS**

General risk factors for violence in such patients include:
- Prior arrests
- Substance abuse
- Presence of hallucinations, delusions, or bizarre behaviors
- Presence of neurological impairment
- Being male, poor, unskilled, uneducated, or unmarried

In addition, more specific risk factors include:
- Young age
- High IQ
- High level of premorbid scholastic achievement
- High aspirations
- Insight, awareness into illness and losses
- Chronic intermittent course characterized by relapses and exacerbations of illness

TABLE 8-2 CATEGORIES OF VIOLENCE-PRONE DISORDERS

Psychosis	• In the community, paranoid schizophrenics are more violent than other diagnostic categories; in the hospital, nonparanoid patients are more likely to be violent • Paranoid patients with delusions may be at higher risk to commit a violent act because of their ability to plan and their retention of some reality testing • Directed at specific person seen as persecuting the patient (relatives, friend) • Weapon use because of access
Personality disorder	Traits associated with violence: • Impulsivity • Low frustration tolerance • Inability to tolerate criticism • Egocentricity and entitlement • Tendency to have superficial relationships and to dehumanize others • Glib, lack of introspection, tendency to externalize blame • Failure to accept responsibility for one's actions Psychopathic traits include: • Cold, lack of empathy • Lack of remorse
Dementia	• Impaired executive functioning • Increased agitation • Sometimes hallucinations and/or delusions
Mania	• More likely to be assaultive without prior threats although often respond violently to any limit setting • 26% of patients with mania attack someone within the first 24 hours of hospitalization
Depression	• Despair, in rare cases, could lead to striking out against other people • Murder-suicide is suicide within 1 week of a homicide; in couples it is highly associated with jealousy • The individual can no longer endure a life without what is perceived to be a vital element (e.g., a spouse, family, job, health) but cannot bear the thought of the other persons carrying on without him, so he forces the others to join him in death. Always ask a suicidal mother about her children.
GMC	• Disinhibition, irritability, psychosis
Premenstrual dysphoric disorder	• Anxiety, tension, irritability, hypersensitivity
PTSD	• Anxiety, hypervigilance • Reactive to external cues

TABLE 8-3 SPECIFIC PSYCHOTIC SYMPTOMS THAT MAY BE ASSOCIATED WITH INCREASED RISK OF VIOLENCE

Command hallucinations	• Specific instructions to commit: • Suicide—52% • Homicide—5% • Injury to self or others—12% • Nonviolent acts—14% Compliance to command hallucinations: • Wide range—10–80% • Reduced if command is dangerous • Increased with a hallucination-related delusion (double distortion of reality) • Increased if voice is familiar • Reduced in an inpatient setting
Delusions	• The majority of persons with schizophrenia experience delusions during their illness Violence is more likely if delusions: • Are systematized • Are preceded by fear or anger • Were acted on before • Are coupled with substance abuse • Are of being persecuted or poisoned • Delusional misidentification, (e.g., Capgras' syndrome) is the most common in which a patient believes that others have been replaced by physical duplicates who have different psychological identities from the original • Erotomanic—More common in males than females but less than 5% commit a violent act and sometimes that is committed toward one who is perceived as standing in the way of the loved one (e.g., wife, bodyguard) • *Threat control override (TCO) symptoms were found to be associated with increased aggression:* • *Mind feels dominated by forces beyond individual's control* • *Feelings that thoughts are being put into your head* • *People wish you harm* • *Belief that you are being followed*

Note: The MacArthur study did NOT support this conclusion about TCO delusions.

	Delusions not associated with increased aggression: • Feeling dead, dissolved, or not existing • Feeling that your thoughts are broadcast • Feelings that thoughts are taken by external force
GMC	• Neuropsychological deficits • Traumatic brain injury • Intermittent explosive disorder • Seizure disorder

WORKING WITH SECURITY AND POLICE

The twenty-first century urban psychiatric emergency service (PES), such as that found in the authors' respective workplaces, typically has a security system in place. Prior to entering the PES, a patient arrives at an outside entrance area where he/she must pass through a metal/weapons detector. A security officer conducts a search of the prospective patient similar to that experienced by airport travelers. In the authors' collective experiences, an array of interesting and frightening weapons have been collected, from crudely fashioned knives to handguns.

Many patients are brought to the PES by police officers; often the officers bring a patient in handcuffs after being called to a private home or finding the individual wandering in traffic. Most of the interactions the authors have had with officers have been overwhelmingly positive with the officers exhibiting professionalism and sensitivity. True, police officers may view the mentally ill patient as an interruption to the flow of their day; they are often eager to drop such a patient off at the PES and be on their way as quickly as possible. This is understandable, but not always acceptable for PES staff. Ideally police officers should remain with the agitated, potentially violent patient while staff medicate the patient and take the patient out of handcuffs and into mechanical restraints. Once this transition is complete, paperwork (if necessary) is filled out (i.e., involuntary commitment forms), and a modicum of calm exists, the officers can safely leave the PES. Ideally this could be accomplished quickly depending on several factors, especially how busy the PES is when the officers arrive.

PES staff need to remember that police officers are trained to quickly subdue someone who is violent toward them or other citizens. When police officers work with mentally ill patients, they put on a different hat; depending on the individual officer and his/her level of training and experience, this may be professionally counterintuitive. The authors have repeatedly seen staff get frustrated with police officers "dropping off patients" and with security "not showing up" to help with out-of-control patients. The PES is a community service and staff need to figure out ways to work effectively and professionally with police officers and internal security forces. The authors advocate for liaison and education as helpful in increasing cooperativeness between law enforcement and PES. The University of Cincinnati PES runs a mobile crisis service and also posts mobile crisis workers in police districts for educational, liaison, and consultative roles for police officers. This has greatly increased the spirit of cooperation between the PES and police in Cincinnati.

PES staff need security; the PES at Temple University, one of the busiest on the East Coast, has full-time security posted in the PES. Their physical presence is crucial to running a fast-paced university-based urban PES. In addition, Temple PES has panic alarms throughout the unit; some PES settings offer personal alarms for staff. Often security or police presence is enough to bring order to a situation. Most are conscientious and have the same goals in the acute phase: to quickly and safely bring order to a situation.

MANAGEMENT OF THE ACUTE POTENTIALLY VIOLENT PATIENT

A 28-year-old male patient is brought in by police yelling, rambling nonsensically; his mother, with whom he lives, has filed for involuntary commitment on the basis of her schizophrenic son stopping his medication a month ago, becoming psychotic (e.g., he believes his mother is trying to poison his food), and his threatening behavior toward her.

The importance of a calm, confident clinical demeanor with attention to one's internal cues (aka countertransference) cannot be overemphasized. Fear is designed to protect us and should be heeded. Approach such a patient cautiously with security at your side. Introduce yourself. Ask a couple of easy questions ("What's your name?" "Do you know where you are now?") to test whether the patient can answer basic orientation questions. Size up the situation quickly ("eyeball" the patient: figure out which major diagnostic category seems most likely, i.e., mood/anxiety/psychotic/substance/personality disorder) and determine what the immediate intervention should be (IM or PO medication, mechanical restraints). It may be possible to verbally de-escalate this situation and, if it looks possible, try to do so without medication. However, bear in mind that your goal is to help this patient regain homeostasis. In the case of the patient above, he spit at staff, could not answer basic orientation questions, and was agitated and internally preoccupied. He calmed with IM psychotropic medication and a brief restraint period. It is often necessary to utilize psychotropic medication to target the psychotic and behavioral agitation symptoms and regain homeostasis as quickly as possible.

Often patients become agitated during their stays in the waiting area or during the interview process. Clinicians should *not hesitate* to leave the interview room or to hit the panic button or personal alarm at the first inclination that the patient may become violent. Do trust your instincts. Do not put yourself in harm's way. Ask for help. For those working in community mental health centers, this is even more crucial. After all, PES staff are trained to deal with such patients and have infrastructures and/or systemic responses in place for just such patients. As a fellow in forensic psychiatry, one of the authors was regularly among inmates in a variety of correctional settings. But it was in a community mental health setting that she felt the most at risk for violence when a large female patient began to stare her down after a relatively innocuous comment. The only other individual in the room was the slightly built case manager, and there was no mechanism to access help (the orientation directive to "pick up the phone and call the front desk for coffee" as a way to discreetly initiate help seemed woefully inadequate and laborious in an actual emergency situation).

If you are interviewing a patient, when you enter the interview room, decide where you think it is safest to seat yourself. Pay attention to your countertransference. If you think it is possible that the patient could become physically violent toward you, seat yourself at the door for quick egress. You will do no good to anyone if you are injured. Take pains to protect yourself. Some repeat patients known to be violent have a little tag on the chart indicating so. Be aware of this. Past violent behavior predicts future violent behavior.

Should a patient become angry during the interview, the clinician can encourage the verbal expression of anger. Encourage the patient to talk about what is bothering him; you don't have to agree particularly if it is delusionally driven. Encourage him to calm himself and offer food or medication to help calm him (Table 8-4).

Many of the PES staff run internal staff training or work with local consultants sensitive to issues specific to the PES or community mental health centers. For example, the Temple PES is located in a predominantly Latino population. We must be sensitive to language barriers and understand what interventions may be more effective with our population vs. a suburban PES setting. In addition, there are institutes that offer professional staff training.

TABLE 8-4 STAY COOL RECOMMENDED CLINICAL DEMEANOR TOWARD THE POTENTIALLY VIOLENT PATIENT

S	**Stand** at a safe distance; 1–2 × arm's length. Positioning oneself side by side rather than face to face with the patient may help the patient see the clinician as less of a foe.
T	**Talk** with an even, concerned voice **tone;** consider **timing** of questions and directives.
A	**Ask** simple questions initially designed to increase rapport; **avoid** being provocative; **agree** to disagree. **Alarms**—know where they are located, how to activate them, and what is expected to happen upon activation.
Y	**Yellow**—do *not* worry about being called a **yellowbelly**. If you feel afraid, get out of the room, away from the situation, and call for help. Better to be slightly embarrassed than beaten up.
C	**Concise.** Don't get long-winded with agitated patients. Keep it simple and repeat yourself as necessary.
O	**Observational** awareness. This is a key part of the skill set of an emergency clinician. Be vigilant for emotional and behavioral cues. Patients usually give warning of impending violence such as pacing, talking to themselves, belligerence toward staff, demanding, entitled demeanor, and not following staff directives. Pay attention to what is going on in the milieu.
O	**Options**—Offer options about treatment and hope for the patient's future. In the immediate situation, the options may be limited, but to offer oral vs. IM medication is to present the patient with an option. **Offer** food, the universal language of hospitality.
L	**Look** and **listen.** Be respectful. Making eye contact is important, but don't get into a staring contest with a potentially aggressive patient. Look off to the side and up; keep your expression neutral. It's obvious who "controls" the clinical situation and it isn't necessary to get into a contest with the patient to prove it. Find out what the patient truly wants and then you can help determine whether that is reasonable or, if not, what can be offered.

VIOLENCE RISK ASSESSMENT

Remember that your primary goal in the emergency situation is to keep the patient safe and to arrive at rapid stabilization and disposition of the patient. To that end, your violence risk assessment should be brief, focused, and encompass information about the current situation and the most prudent way to reduce risk of violence in the here and now. More comprehensive risk assessment is the purview of inpatient care if needed.

Comprehensive violence risk assessment is beyond the scope of this chapter.

Be aware that patients will likely seek to deny or minimize their violence. They typically deny or minimize:

- Use of violence to solve interpersonal problems
- Perceiving oneself as dangerous
- Violent fantasies and dreams
- Violent friends
- Substance abuse
- Hostility
- Past multiple violence
- Institutional conduct involving threats of violence
- Assaults of threats to authority figures
- Arrests and hospitalizations for violence
- Dangerous weapon used in offense
- Possession or recent purchase of firearms
- High hostility, low frustration tolerance
- Chronic anger toward others

However, often these same persons will likely acknowledge the following:

- Convictions
- Prison incarcerations
- Body tattoos with violent theme
- Preference for violent films
- Physical abuse as a child
- Violent role model in the home

Often the patient tries to portray himself as dangerous in the past, but not now. Thus the need for a high index of suspicion and the use of collateral contacts and information.

While actuarial tools may be helpful, the emergency situation calls for a checklist (see Table 8-5) to inform and shape the clinician's thinking in determining whether the individual patient before him or her requires inpatient vs. outpatient care. The clinician is cautioned to utilize the checklist flexibly with the understanding that such a tool is meant to guide a systematic assessment of violence risk (see also Table 8-6). For additional interview questions see Table 8-7.

All threats should be taken seriously and the details should be elucidated.

How well planned is the threat? Consider the following exchange:

Patient: I'm going to go to my ex-wife's apartment and blow her off the face of the earth.
Clinician: How are you going to do this?
Patient: I've got a rifle in the trunk of my car, some trashbags, and a saw. I'm going to shoot her, then dismember her body and pack it into trashbags and throw her in the Ohio River by cover of darkness.
Clinician: This sounds like a well-thought-out plan. I'd like to hospitalize you for a few days to sort this out.

In the case of a paranoid patient, ask what the patient would do if confronted by the perceived persecutor.

Clinician: OK, so you say that people in black raincoats are following you. What would you do if you encountered a person in a black raincoat walking toward you on the street?
Patient: I'd take out my handgun that I keep strapped to my leg and shoot him or maybe I'd run across the street.

Both answers inform the clinical decision-making process. But if the clinician does not ask the question, he/she might not elicit the data that would help in making the best dispositional decision.

Other behaviors associated with paranoid fear to inquire about:

- Changes of residence
- Long trips to evade persecutor
- Barricading one's room
- Carrying weapons for protection
- Asking police for protection

TABLE 8-5 **ASSESSMENT OF VIOLENCE RISK FACTORS**

	Inhibiting	Facilitating
Historical		
Age	_____	_____
Sex	_____	_____
Race	_____	_____
Marital status	_____	_____
Socioeconomic status	_____	_____
Education	_____	_____
IQ	_____	_____
History of childhood arrest	_____	_____
Family history of violence	_____	_____
School failure	_____	_____
Employment status	_____	_____
History of previous violence	_____	_____
Clinical		
Antisocial personality disorder	_____	_____
Axis I primary psychiatric disorder	_____	_____
Axis I substance use disorder	_____	_____
Motivation for treatment	_____	_____
Adherence to treatment regimen	_____	_____
Situational		
Current relationship status	_____	_____
Current living situation	_____	_____
Current legal status	_____	_____
Current exposure/susceptibility to destabilizers (e.g., negative peer pressure, access to drugs)	_____	_____

SOURCE: Adapted from Simon (1997).

TABLE 8-6   **DEMOGRAPHICS OF VIOLENCE**

Age	Violence peaks in the late teens and early 20s
Sex	Males more than females in general population; among people with mental disorders males and females do not significantly differ in their base rates of violence
Social class	Violence is three times as likely in lowest SES than in the highest
Race	The incidence of homicide for a black male is 1 in 21
	The incidence of homicide for a white male is 1 in 131
IQ	The lower, the more violence
History of substance abuse	Substance abuse tripled the rate of violence in the nonpatients in the community and increased the rate of violence by discharged patients by up to five times
Education	Less education
Employment	Lack of sustained employment
Residential instability	Homeless mentally ill commit 35 times more crimes than domiciled mentally ill
Diagnosis	• The higher the number of psychiatric diagnoses, the greater the rate of violence • The combination of substance abuse with other major psychopathy is more volatile than either alone • At least one-third of patients with schizophrenia also meet criteria for substance use disorder

TABLE 8-7   **WEAPONS HISTORY ASSESSMENT**

• Have you ever owned a weapon?
• What kind(s)?
• Do you own any now?
• What do you do with the weapons? Where do you keep them? Are they loaded?
• Have you moved the weapon lately? (This is a tipoff of imminent risk.)
• Did you ever threaten, injure, or kill a person(s) with a weapon?

OVERT AGGRESSION SCALE (TABLE 8-8)

This scale was developed by Yudofsky and colleagues, is reliable, and is helpful in measuring the following parameters:

- Verbal aggression against staff, other people, and objects
- Physical aggression against staff, other people, and objects
- Degree of seriousness, injury, or damage of above
- Duration and timing of aggression
- Types of intervention

TABLE 8-8 THE OVERT AGGRESSION SCALE

Name of patient _____ Sex of patient _____

Name of rater _____

Date _____

Shift _____

Aggressive behavior (check all that apply)

Verbal aggression

_____ Makes loud noises, shouts angrily

_____ Yells mild personal insults (e.g., "You're stupid")

_____ Curses viciously, uses foul language in anger, makes moderate threats to others or self

_____ Makes clear threats of violence toward others or self (e.g., "I'm going to kill you") or requests help to control self

Physical aggression against objects

_____ Slams door, scatters clothing, makes a mess

_____ Throws objects down, kicks furniture without breaking it, marks the wall

_____ Breaks objects, smashes windows

_____ Sets fires, throws objects dangerously

Physical aggression against self

_____ Picks or scratches skin, hits self, pulls hair (with no or minor head injury only)

_____ Bangs head, hits fist into objects, throws self onto floor or into objects (hurts self without serious injury)

_____ Small cuts or bruises, minor burns

_____ Mutilates self, makes deep cuts, bites that bleed, internal injury, fracture, loss of consciousness, loss of teeth

Physical aggression against other people

_____ Makes threatening gestures, swings at people, grabs at clothes

_____ Strikes, kicks, pushes, pulls hair (without injury to them)

_____ Attacks others, causing mild or moderate physical injury (bruises, sprain, welts)

_____ Attacks others, causing severe physical injury (broken bones, deep lacerations, internal injury)

Time incident began: _____ Duration: _____

Intervention: _____

Response to intervention: _____

SOURCE: Adapted from Yudofsky SC, et al. The Overt Aggression Scale for the Objective Rating of Verbal and Physical Aggression. *American Journal of Psychiatry* 143 (1986): 35–39.

LEGAL ISSUES IN THE PREDICTION OF VIOLENCE

The Tarasoff case involved the violent death of a University of California at Berkeley coed named Tatiana Tarasoff. The man who murdered her was a fellow student named Prosenjitt Poddar; after he was romantically rejected by Tarasoff, Poddar began counseling sessions with a University psychologist. In the course of therapy, Poddar admitted to homicidal feelings toward Tarasoff. The psychologist called campus police to involuntarily hospitalize Poddar; instead, they inexplicably released him. Within months, Poddar killed Tarasoff. The Tarasoff family brought a civil suit against the University psychologist and staff for failure to warn them of the risk to their daughter. This resulted in Tarasoff I, the duty to warn; Tarasoff II, the duty to protect (Table 8-9); and subsequent Tarasoff progeny. Most states have addressed the mental health professional's duty to warn or protect either in case law or by statute and the reader is advised to be familiar with his/her state's position on this issue.

This is not an unusual situation in the PES. If the patient is deemed at risk of harming an innocent third party, has specified the third party, and has specified the means of carrying out the threat, hospitalization is recommended. The authors' experience is that such a patient needs a few days to "cool the blood" and, after he has done so, the crisis resolves and the patient is able to formulate a plan to deal with his anger at the third party. In unresolved situations in which the patient remains persistently homicidal, a more detailed violence risk assessment with risk reduction recommendations/interventions may be warranted. Such violence risk assessments are often completed by forensic psychiatrists.

TABLE 8-9 TARASOFF II: THE DUTY TO PROTECT

"When a therapist determines, or, according to the standard of his profession, should determine, that his patient presents a serious danger of violence to another, he incurs an obligation to use reasonable care to protect the intended victim from danger." This duty may be discharged as follows:

- Warn the intended victim
- Warn others who will apprise the victim
- Notify police
- Hospitalize the patient

SUICIDE RISK IN PERSONS MAKING HOMICIDAL THREATS

It is well worth noting the following facts:

- In the United States, 4% of homicides also involve suicide.
- Violent suicide attempts increase the likelihood of future violence toward others. Nonviolent suicide attempts (e.g., by overdose or carbon monoxide) do not.
- In a 1997 study, 91% of outpatients who had attempted homicide also had attempted suicide, and 86% of patients with homicidal ideation also reported suicidal ideation.

RISK MANAGEMENT STRATEGIES

- Be as thorough and systematic as possible in evaluating patients in the PES setting. Utilize a checklist to guide your professional judgment and document well.
- Documentation should include the dispositional decision made (inpatient, outpatient) and the specifics of how the clinical decision was made, including the data used to make the decision. It is not unreasonable to show your clinical thinking process on paper (e.g., "I considered option A, but chose option B for the following reasons"). Note how your dispositional choice was arrived at (i.e., with the patient's participation or without). Comment on the therapeutic rapport between yourself and the patient. As with suicide risk assessment, your patient's safety, the safety of others, and your own liability risk will all be improved with a thorough assessment versus a signed "no-harm" contract.
- Courts are likely to be more sympathetic to the clinician who completes a thorough assessment that informs a well-thought-out plan, but a "bad outcome," than to the clinician with a poor evaluation. There are inherent limitations in the PES setting (time constraints, difficulty in obtaining records) and courts should recognize this.
- Regular, updated, staff training is crucial. In a study of psychiatric residents, their perception of PES staff as competent was the factor that most bolstered their sense of safety in the psychiatric emergency setting.

BIBLIOGRAPHY

Allen MH, Currier GW, Hughes DH, Reyes-Harde M, Docherty JP. The Expert Consensus Guideline Series. Treatment of Behavioral Emergencies. *Postgraduate Medicine* (May 2001) (Spec No): 1–88; quiz 89–90.

Appelbaum PS, Robbins PC, Monahan J. Violence and Delusions: Data from the MacArthur Violence Risk Assessment Study. *American Journal of Psychiatry* 157(4) (April 2000): 566–72.

Binder RL, McNiel DE. Emergency Psychiatry: Contemporary Practices in Managing Acutely Violent Patients in 20 Psychiatric Emergency Rooms. *Psychiatric Services* 50(12) (1999): 1553–54.

Black KJ, Compton WM, Wetzel M, Minchin S, Farber NB, Rastogi-Cruz D. Assaults by Patients on Psychiatric Residents at Three Training Sites. *Hospital Community Psychiatry* 45(7) (July 1994): 706–10.

Busch AB, Shore MF. Seclusion and Restraint: A Review of Recent Literature. *Harvard Review of Psychiatry* 8(5) (November 2000): 261–70.

Coontz PD, Lidz CW, Mulvey EP. Gender and the Assessment of Dangerousness in the Psychiatric Emergency Room. *Internal Journal of Law and Psychiatry* 17(4) (Fall 1994): 369–76.

de Becker G. *The Gift of Fear.* New York: Dell Publishing, 1997.

Diagnostic and Statistical Manual of Mental Disorders, 4th ed., Text Revision (DSM-IV-TR). Washington, DC: American Psychiatric Association, 2000.

Dolan M, Doyle M. Violence Risk Prediction. Clinical and Actuarial Measures and the Role of the Psychopathy Checklist. *British Journal of Psychiatry* 177 (2000): 303–11.

Felthous AR, Hempel A. Combined Homicide-Suicides: A Review. *Journal of Forensic Sciences* 40 (1995): 846–57.

Fishkind A. Calming Agitation with Words, not Drugs. *Current Psychiatry* 1(4) (2002): 32–40.

Flannery RB Jr, Walker AP. Safety Skills of Mental Health Workers: Empirical Evidence of a Risk Management Strategy. *Psychiatric Quarterly* 74(1) (Spring 2003): 1–10.

Herbert PB, Young KA. Tarasoff at Twenty-five. *Journal of American Academy of Psychiatry and Law* 30(2) (2002): 275–81.

Hughes DH. Suicide and Violence Assessment in Psychiatry. *General Hospital Psychiatry* 18(6) (November 1996): 416–21.

Martell DA, et al. Base Rate Estimates of Criminal Behavior by Homeless Mentally Ill Persons in New York City. *Psychiatric Services* 46 (1995): 596–601.

Mason T. Gender Differences in the Use of Seclusion. *Medical Science and Law* 38(1) (January 1998): 2–9.

McNeil DE, Eisner JP, Binder RL. The Relationship between Command Hallucinations Mental Disorders. *Psychiatric Services* 51(10) (October 2000): 1288–92.

Monahan J, et al. *Rethinking Risk Assessment: The MacArthur Study of Mental Disorder and Violence.* New York: Oxford University Press, 2001.

Nestor PG. Mental Disorder and Violence: Personality Dimensions and Clinical Features. *American Journal of Psychiatry* 159(12) (December 2002): 1973–78.

Resnick PJ. Violence Risk Assessment. AAPL Forensic Psychiatry Review Course, 2002.

Silver E, Mulvey EP, Monahan J. Assessing Violence Risk among Discharged Psychiatric Patients: Toward an Ecological Approach. *Law and Human Behavior* 23(2) (April 1999): 237–55.

Simon RI. *Concise Guide to Psychiatry and Law for Clinicians*, 3rd ed. Washington, DC: American Psychiatric Publishing, 2001, 179–214.

Skeem JL, Mulvey EP. Psychopathy and Community Violence Among Civil Psychiatric Patients: Results from the MacArthur Violence Risk Assessment Study. *Journal of Consulting Clinical Psychology* 69(3) (June 2001): 358–74.

Southcott J, Howard A, Collins E. Control and Restraint Training in Acute Mental Health Care. *Nursing Standards* 16(27) (March 20–26, 2002): 33–36.

Yudofsky SC, et al. The Overt Aggression Scale for the Objective Rating of Verbal and Physical Aggression. *American Journal of Psychiatry* 143 (1986): 35–39.

Chapter 9

MOOD/ANXIETY DISORDERS

INTRODUCTION

Mood and anxiety disorders are among the most prevalent of psychiatric disorders. Often patients present in a crisis due to a panic attack or family members may bring a severely depressed and psychotic family member to a community mental health clinic for care. Both disorders are eminently treatable, but without treatment, the risk of associated syndromes and premature death by suicide is high, (i.e., up to 15% of individuals with severe MDD die by suicide and 10–15% of individuals with bipolar illness die by suicide). Anxiety disorders also have a high prevalence in the general population and have significant comorbidity and risk of premature death.

The goals of this chapter include:

1. Review definitions
2. Review DSM-IV-TR diagnostic criteria for mood disorders in a table format that elucidates prevalence/core symptoms/associated symptoms/course/differential diagnosis; address culture-age-gender considerations
3. Review DSM-IV-TR diagnostic criteria for anxiety disorders in a table format that elucidates prevalence/core symptoms/associated symptoms/course/differential diagnosis; address culture-age-gender considerations
4. Review biopsychosocial treatment options briefly and provide algorithms for differential diagnosis and treatment of mood/anxiety disorders

DEFINITIONS

1. Mood is defined as the internal typical state of an individual ("the climate")
2. Affect is defined as the external manifestation of mood ("the weather")

    Mood Disorders are divided into the following categories:

    - Depressive disorders—distinguished from bipolar disorders by the fact that there is no history of ever having a manic, hypomanic, or mixed episode
    - Bipolar disorders
    - Mood disorder due to a general medical condition (GMC)
    - Substance-induced mood disorder

3. Anxiety is defined as the free-floating sense of dread often without any sense of a specific source although typically it is triggered by anticipation and/or experience of a specific object, situation, or event

    Anxiety Disorders are divided into the following:

    - Panic disorder
    - Panic disorder with agoraphobia
    - Panic disorder without agoraphobia
    - Generalized anxiety disorder (GAD)
    - Social phobia
    - Simple phobias
    - Subtypes include
        - Environmental
        - Animal
        - Situational
    - Obsessive compulsive disorder (OCD)
    - Posttraumatic stress disorder (PTSD)
    - Anxiety disorder due to a GMC
    - Substance-induced anxiety disorder
    - Anxiety disorder NOS

It isn't often that a patient presents with a tidy laundry list of DSM-IV-TR diagnostic criteria. A patient is a human being with a unique personality style and is likely to present in a myriad of ways.

The authors view the emergency presentation as a phasic one with the emergency as the initial phase. At this point it is most relevant to accurately place the patient into a diagnostic category (Figure 9-1). The categories are broad and include mood disorders, anxiety disorders, psychotic/schizophrenia disorders, substance abuse, and personality disorders. There is often overlap: individuals may, and often do, fit into a multitude of categories.

Risk factors for suicide are covered in Chapter 7, "The Potentially Suicidal Patient."

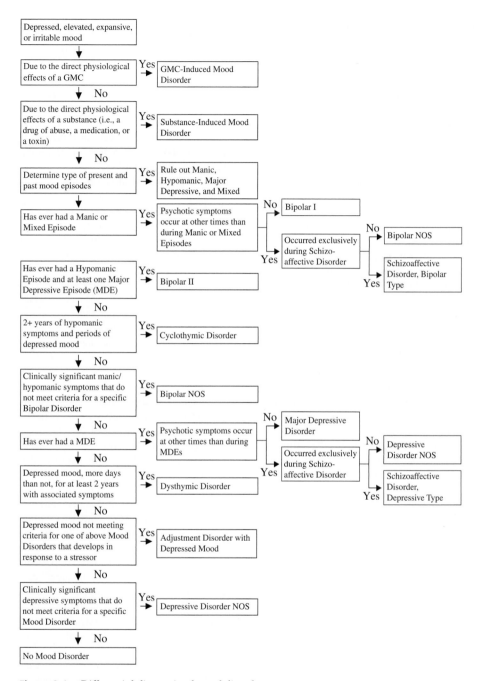

Figure 9-1 *Differential diagnosis of mood disorders.*

Source: Adapted from *Diagnostic and Statistical Manual of Mental Disorders*, 4th ed., Text Revision (Washington, DC: American Psychiatric Association, 2000) (hereafter DSM-IV-TR), pp. 752–53.

DEPRESSIVE DISORDERS

The depressive disorders include major depression with various degrees of severity from mild to moderate to severe with or without psychosis. Further classification is based on subtype (Table 9-1). Such diagnostic specifics help to predict treatment response and specific treatments that may be the most helpful.

The types of depressive mood disorders are described in Tables 9-2 to 9-7.

1. Depression in children and adolescents may manifest very different from that in adults. For example, a teenage boy who presents with conduct problems and aggression may be suffering from an underlying mood disorder or a child whose grades have dropped may be experiencing concentration problems associated with depression.
2. Depression in the elderly may be seen as not eating and forgetfulness. It is important to distinguish between depression and dementia and/or medical illness. Diagnostic clues include:
   a. The elderly patient complains of forgetfulness rather than trying to cover it up or hide it. This can be important in distinguishing a cognitive disorder from a depression with associated decreased concentration, confusion or difficulty thinking, and decreased energy. It is important to not be dismissive of the older adult with medical illnesses as "just being tired" from the illness or because they are "just old."
   b. A history of an older adult with a typically bright energetic demeanor who becomes withdrawn and isolative, crying, etc., strongly suggests the need to investigate for depression and to rule out medical etiologies.
3. Depression in Women. With postpartum depression it is crucial to rule out a more serious postpartum psychosis and/or to prevent the patient from developing a postpartum psychosis. Postpartum blues are common, occurring in up to 70% of women during the first 10 days postpartum, are transient, and do not impair functioning. Postpartum mood episodes with psychosis occur in from 1 in 500 to 1 in 1000 deliveries. Infanticide is most often associated with postpartum psychotic episodes that are characterized by command hallucinations to kill the infant or delusions that the infant is possessed, but it can also occur in severe postpartum mood episodes without such specific hallucinations or delusions.

   A major risk of discontinuing medications after conception is recurrence of depression. This may have a negative impact on fetal development, such as low birth weight or preterm delivery. Factors to consider include the woman's history of depression (e.g., number and severity of prior episodes, degree of functional impairment during episodes in a woman currently taking antidepressants who is either attempting to conceive or is newly pregnant, and the severity of depression in a woman who is currently off medications and is pregnant).

   The emergency clinician should be aware of the typical course of depression and anxiety because of his educative role to patients. Women are twice as likely to experience depression than men, with a lifetime prevalence of 10–25%. Women are most at risk during their childbearing years (onset of depression peaks in women between 25 and 44 years of age). Thus in an emergency setting it is most likely that clinicians will be seeing a population of women in this age range—in other words women who may be trying to conceive, are pregnant, or postpartum. Because ethical considerations preclude prospective, randomized controlled trials that would pose danger to the fetus or newborn, physicians must rely on observational studies in making treatment decisions in this area.
4. Cultural considerations in depression. Cultural differences exist in presentations of depression. Culture can influence the experience and communication of symptoms of depression. For example, in some cultures,

depression may be experienced largely in somatic terms.

- Complaints of nerves and headaches (Latino and Mediterranean)
- Weakness, tiredness, or imbalance (Chinese or Asian)

- Problems of the heart (Middle Eastern)
- Heartbroken (Hopi)

Cultures may also differ in judgments about the seriousness of experiencing or expressing dysphoria.

TABLE 9-1   **SPECIFIERS FOR MOOD DISORDERS**

Current clinical status and/or features	Mild, moderate, severe without psychotic features/severe with psychotic features
Features of the most recent episode	With catatonic features
	With melancholic features
	With atypical features
	With postpartum onset
Longitudinal course specifiers	With and without interepisode recovery
	With seasonal pattern

SOURCE: Adapted from DSM-IV-TR, pp. 346–47.

TABLE 9-2 **MAJOR DEPRESSIVE DISORDER (MDD)**

Prevalence and familial pattern	10–25% women 5–12% men 1.5–3 times more common among first-degree biological relatives Up to 20–25% of individuals with certain GMCs will develop an MDD during the course of their GMC
Core symptoms	Characterized by one or more major depressive episodes, (i.e., at least 2 weeks of depressed mood or loss of interest accompanied by at least 4 additional symptoms of depression)
Associated symptoms	Can present with: • Tearfulness • Irritability • Brooding • Excessive rumination • Anxiety, sometimes even meeting criteria for panic disorder • Phobias • Excessive worry over physical health • Complaints of pain • Difficulty in intimate relationships • Difficulties in sexual function • Marital problems • Occupational problems • Academic problems • Comorbid substance abuse • Increased utilization of medical services • Most serious consequence can be attempted or completed suicide Up to 15% of individuals with severe MDD die by suicide
Course	Symptoms develop over days to weeks, (i.e., a prodrome of anxiety and mild depression may last for weeks to months before the onset of a full MDD) If untreated, 4 months or longer In a majority of cases, complete remission of symptoms and functioning returns to premorbid level Preceded by Dysthymic Disorder in 10% of epidemiological samples and 15–25% of clinical samples Each year approximately 10% of individuals with Dysthymic Disorder alone will go on to have a first MDD Course is variable average age of onset is mid-20s The number of prior episodes predicts the likelihood of developing subsequent Major DE 60% of individuals with MDD, Single Episode, will have a second episode, individuals who have had 2 episodes have a 70% chance of having a third, and individuals who have had 3 episodes have a 90% chance of having a fourth About 5–10% of individuals with MDD Single Episode subsequently develop a manic episode

(continued)

TABLE 9-2   **MAJOR DEPRESSIVE DISORDER (MDD)—Continued**

	May end completely in two-thirds of cases, partially, or not at all; those who experience partial remission have a greater likelihood of developing an additional episode and of continuing the pattern of partial interepisode recovery
Differential diagnosis	*Mood disorder due to a GMC*: if the mood disturbance is judged to be the direct physiological consequence of a specific GMC. Base this on history, lab findings, and/or physical exam. Both can be present (i.e., if the MDD is a psychological consequence of having the GMC or there is no etiological relationship between the MDD and the medical condition)
	Substance-induced mood disorder
	Dementia in elderly: by thorough medical evaluation; evaluate the onset of the disturbance, temporal sequencing of depressive and cognitive symptoms, course of illness, and treatment response.
	Premorbid state: in dementia there is usually a premorbid history of declining cognitive functions whereas the individual with MDD will have a normal premorbid function and rapid decline of cognitive function associated with the MDD
	Manic Episodes with irritable mood or mixed episodes
	ADHD in children may be present with distractibility and low frustration tolerance
	Adjustment with depressed mood: i.e., full criteria are not met for MDD
	Bereavement after the loss of a loved one unless the symptoms persist for more than 2 months or include marked functional impairment, morbid preoccupation with worthlessness, suicidal ideation, psychotic symptoms, or psychomotor retardation
	Normal periods of sadness
	Depressive disorder NOS may be an appropriate diagnosis for presentations of depressed mood with clinically significant impairment that do not meet criteria for duration or severity

SOURCE: Adapted from DSM-IV-TR, pp. 349–56, 369–76.

TABLE 9-3   DYSTHYMIC DISORDER (DD)

Prevalence and familial pattern	Lifetime prevalence with/without superimposed MDD is 6%. In adulthood, women are 2–3 times more likely to develop dysthymic disorder than are men.
Core symptoms	At least 2 years of depressed mood (1 year for children and adolescents) for more days than not (any symptom-free intervals last no longer than 2 months), accompanied by additional depressive symptoms that do not meet criteria for MDE.
Associated symptoms	Associated features are similar to those of MDE.
Course	Early and insidious onset in childhood, adolescence, or young adulthood. Often those in clinical settings have a superimposed MDD ("double depression"). If dysthymic disorder precedes MDD, there is less likelihood of spontaneous full interepisode recovery between MDSs and a greater likelihood of having more frequent subsequent episodes. The treated course of dysthymic disorder is similar to that of other depressive disorders whether or not there is a superimposed MDD. Vegetative symptoms are less common in dysthymic disorder.
Differential diagnosis	*Mood disorder due to a GMC and a substance-induced mood disorder*, by history, lab findings, and/or physical examinations. If the depressive symptoms are the direct physiological consequence of the GMC or substance use, then no diagnosis of mood disorder. If the symptoms are judged to be the psychological consequence of the GMC, then diagnosis can be made. Coexisting personality disorder may also be present. The diagnosis of dysthymic disorder can be made following a MDD only if the DD was established prior to the first MDE (i.e., no MDE during the first 2 years of dysthymic symptoms or if there has been a full remission of the MDD lasting at least 2 months before the onset of the DD). Depressive symptoms may be commonly associated with *chronic psychotic disorders*. However, a DD diagnosis is not made if the symptoms occur only during the course of the psychotic disorder including residual phases.

SOURCE: Adapted from DSM-IV-TR, pp. 376–81.

TABLE 9-4 **DEPRESSIVE DISORDER NOS**

Coding disorders that do not meet the criteria for MDD, DD, and adjustment disorder or depressive symptoms about which there is inadequate or contradictory information

The following are examples:
- Premenstrual dysphoric disorder
- Minor depressive disorder
- Recurrent brief depressive disorder
- Postpsychotic depressive disorder of schizophrenia
- A major depressive episode superimposed on delusional disorder, psychotic disorder NOS, or the active phase of schizophrenia

Situations in which the clinician has concluded that a depressive disorder is present but is unable to determine whether it is primary, due to a GMC, or substance-induced*

---

*This last criterion is what often makes this diagnostic category particularly appropriate for the emergency psychiatry situation. It is not a "copout" to utilize the NOS category. Rather it is a judicious use of a diagnostic category. Clinicians have an extraordinary power: the power to diagnose. The authors consider it a misuse of that power to inappropriately and prematurely diagnose an individual based on an emergency presentation. It is far wiser to be broad, generate a list of differential diagnoses, and leave it to the inpatient and/or treating psychiatrist to be more diagnostically precise.

SOURCE: Adapted from DSM-IV-TR, pp. 381–82.

TABLE 9-5 **MOOD DISORDER DUE TO A GENERAL MEDICAL CONDITION**

Prevalence and familial pattern	25–40% of individuals with certain neurological conditions (e.g., Parkinson's, Huntington's, MS, stroke, and Alzheimer's disease) will develop a marked depressive disturbance at some point during the course of the illness. More variable for GMCs without direct CNS involvement (i.e., 8% in ESRD and 60% in Cushing's).
Core symptoms	A prominent and persistent disturbance in mood that is judged to be due to the direct physiological effects of a GMC. The mood disturbance may involve depressed mood; markedly diminished interest or pleasure; or elevated, expansive, or irritable mood.
Associated symptoms	Associated physical examination findings, lab findings, and patterns of prevalence or onset reflect the etiological GMC.
Differential diagnosis	*Delirium*: A separate diagnosis of mood disturbance is not made if the mood disturbance occurs exclusively during the course of a delirium. This is in contrast to *dementia*. Both diagnoses can be given if the mood symptoms are a direct etiological consequence of the pathological process causing the dementia and if the mood symptoms are a prominent part of the clinical presentation. The exception to this is if depressive symptoms occur exclusively during the course of vascular dementia. *Substance-Induced Mood Disorder.* If there is evidence of recent or prolonged substance use (including medications with psychoactive effects). Symptoms that occur during or shortly after (i.e., within 4 weeks of substance intoxication or withdrawal or after medication use) may be especially indicative of a substance-induced disorder, depending on the character, duration, or amount of the substance used. If it is determined that the mood disturbance is due to both GMC and substance use, both diagnoses can be given. *MDD, BPI, BPII, and adjustment with depressed mood* (a maladaptive response to having a GMC).

SOURCE: Adapted from DSM-IV-TR, pp. 401–5.

TABLE 9-6 SUBSTANCE-INDUCED MOOD DISORDER

Core symptoms	A prominent and persistent disturbance in mood judged to be due to the direct physiological effects of a substance (drug of abuse, a medication, other somatic treatment for depression, or toxin exposure). The mood disturbance may involve depressed mood; markedly diminished interest or pleasure; or elevated, expansive, or irritable mood.

Mood disorders occur in association with *intoxication* with the following classes of substances:

- Alcohol
- Amphetamine
- Cocaine
- Hallucinogens
- Sedative-hypnotics

Mood disorders occur in association with *withdrawal* with the following classes of substances:
- Alcohol
- Amphetamines
- Cocaine
- Amphetamine
- Opioids

Medications that may evoke mood symptoms include:
- Anesthetics
- Analgesics
- Anticholinergics
- Anticonvulsants
- Antihypertensives
- Antiparkinsonian medication
- Antiulcer medication
- Cardiac medication
- Oral contraceptives
- Psychotropics
- Muscle relaxants
- Steroids
- Sulfonamides
- Reserpine
- Corticosteroids and anabolic steroids have an especially high likelihood of producing depressive features
- Heavy metals and toxins like volatile substances, such as gasoline and paint
- Organophosphate insecticides
- Nerve gases
- Carbon monoxide
- Carbon dioxide

(continued)

TABLE 9-6 SUBSTANCE-INDUCED MOOD DISORDER—Continued

Differential diagnosis	*Primary mood disturbance* by considering the onset, course, and other facts. History, physical exam, and lab findings help to rule out.
	Primary mood disorders may precede the onset of substance use or may occur during times of sustained abstinence.
	The presence of atypical features such as atypical age at onset or course (e.g., the onset of a manic episode after age 45 may suggest a substance-induced etiology).
	Factors that suggest mood symptoms are better accounted for by a primary mood disorder include: Persistence of mood symptoms for a substantial period of time, such as a month or more after the end of substance intoxication or acute substance withdrawal; the development of mood symptoms that are substantially in excess of what would be expected given the type or amount of the substance used or the duration of use; or a history of prior recurrent primary episode of mood disorder.

SOURCE: Adapted from DSM-IV-TR, pp. 405–9.

TABLE 9-7 MOOD DISORDER NOS

	Includes disorders with mood symptoms that do not meet the criteria for any specific mood disorder and in which it is difficult to choose between depressive disorder NOS and bipolar disorder NOS (e.g., acute agitation) if it cannot be determined whether a mood disturbance is primary, substance-induced, or due to a GMC

SOURCE: Adapted from DSM-IV-TR, p. 410.

BIPOLAR DISORDERS

The bipolar disorders include BPI, BPII, cyclothymia, and bipolar disorder NOS. There are also six criteria sets for BPI: single manic episode, most recent episode hypomanic, most recent episode manic, most recent episode mixed, most recent episode depressed, most recent episode unspecified.

There are specifiers to describe the current clinical status of the episode and to describe features of the episode (Table 9-8).

The types of bipolar disorder are described in Tables 9-9 to 9-12.

1. Bipolar disorders in children and adolescents. Approximately 10–15% of adolescents with recurrent major depressive episodes will go on to develop BPI. Mixed episodes are more likely in adolescents and young adults.
2. Bipolar disorders in the elderly. Mixed episodes are less likely in this population.
3. Women and bipolar disorders. Bipolar disorders are equally common in men and women, but while the first episode in men is typically a manic episode, in women it is typically a depressive episode. Major depressive episodes predominate in women. Rapid cycling is more common in women than in men. Women with BPI have an increased risk of developing subsequent episodes in the immediate postpartum period and some have their first episode in the postpartum period. The premenstrual period may be associated with worsening of an ongoing major depressive, manic, mixed, or hypomanc episode.
4. Cultural considerations in bipolar disorders. There are no reports of differential incidence of BPI based on race or ethnicity.

Combined medication and psychotherapy is the standard treatment for severe depression. Psychotherapy—cognitive behavioral therapy (CBT) and interpersonal psychotherapy (IPT)—alone has traditionally been recommended for the treatment of mild depression.

The biopsychosocial treatment of mood disorders is outlined in Table 9-13.

TABLE 9-8 BIPOLAR DISORDER SPECIFIERS

Severity	Mild, moderate, severe without psychotic features, severe with psychotic features
Features	With catatonic features
	With postpartum onset
Longitudinal course	With or without full interepisode recovery
	With seasonal pattern
	With rapid cycling

Source: Adapted from DSM-IV-TR, pp. 382–83.

TABLE 9-9 BIPOLAR I

Prevalence and familial pattern	Lifetime prevalence in community samples is 0.4–1.6%.
	Twin and adoption studies provide strong evidence of a genetic influence for BPI.
	First-degree biological relatives of individuals with BPI have elevated rates of BPI (4–24%), BPII (1–5%), and MDD (4–24%).
	Individuals with mood disorder in their first-degree biological relatives are more likely to have an earlier age at onset.

(continued)

TABLE 9-9   BIPOLAR I—Continued

Core symptoms	The essential feature is a clinical course that is characterized by the occurrence of one or more manic episodes or mixed episodes.
Associated symptoms	Violent behavior School truancy, occupational failure Divorce Episodic antisocial behavior Alcohol and substance abuse Particularly if earlier onset of BP
Course	Average age of onset is 20 years for both women and men. Recurrent disorder; more than 90% of individuals who have a single manic episode go on to have future episodes. Intervals between episodes decrease as the individual ages. 5–15% of individuals with BPI have 4 or more mood episodes within a given year, have a rapid cycling pattern, associated with a poorer prognosis. Completed suicide occurs in 10–15%.
Differential diagnosis	*Mood disorder due to a GMC and substance-induced mood disorder* Again, based on history, laboratory findings, and or physical examination. If a manic or mixed episode is precipitated by antidepressant treatment (medication, ECT, or light therapy), these are considered substance-induced and do not count toward a diagnosis of BPI. However, if the medication or treatment is not determined to fully account for the mood episode, i.e., the episode continues long after the substance is discontinued, it is more likely a primary mood disorder. *MDD and DD* by the lifetime history of at least one manic or mixed episode. *BPII* by the presence of one or more manic or mixed episodes. *Cyclothymic* BPI is distinguished by the presence of one or more manic or mixed episodes. *Psychotic disorders* may be difficult since these disorders may share a number of presenting symptoms such as grandiose and persecutory delusions, irritability, agitation, and catatonic symptoms. *Schizophrenia, schizoaffective disorder, and delusional disorder* are all characterized by periods of psychotic symptoms in the absence of prominent mood symptoms. Also consider the accompanying symptoms, previous course, and family history. Manic and depressive symptoms may be present during schizophrenia, schizoaffective disorder, and delusional disorder but rarely with sufficient number, duration, and pervasiveness to meet criteria for a manic or major depressive episode. *BP NOS diagnosis* can be made in those rare instances when full criteria are met.

SOURCE: Adapted from DSM-IV-TR, pp. 382–92.

TABLE 9-10 **BIPOLAR II**

Prevalence and familial pattern	Lifetime prevalence in community samples is 0.5%. First-degree relatives of individuals with BPII have elevated rates of BPII, BPI, and MDD compared with the general population.
Core symptoms	Essential feature is a clinical course that is characterized by the occurrence of one or more major depressive episodes accompanied by at least one hypomanic episode.
Associated symptoms	Similar to above with BPII. School truancy, school failure, occupational failure, and divorce may be associated with BPII. Associated mental disorders include substance abuse, anorexia nervosa, bulimia, ADHD, panic, social phobia, and BPD.
Course	Roughly 60–70% of the hypomanic episodes in BPII occur immediately before or after a MDE; often hypomanic episodes follow a characteristic pattern for a particular person. Like BPI, the interval between episodes tends to decrease with age. 5–15% of individuals with BPII have a rapid-cycling pattern, associated with a poorer prognosis. The majority of individuals return to fully functional baseline between episodes; approximately 15% continue to display mood liability and interpersonal or occupational difficulties. Over 5 years, about 5–15% of individuals with BPII will develop a manic episode.
Differential diagnosis	*Mood disorder due to a GMC substance-induced mood disorder MDD*, by the lifetime history of at least one hypomanic episode. Attention during the interview to whether there is a history of euphoric or dysphoric hypomanic behavior is important in making a differential diagnosis. BPII is distinguished from *BPI* by the presence of one or more manic or mixed episodes in the latter. In *cyclothymic* disorder, there are numerous periods of hypomanic and numerous periods of depressive symptoms that do not meet symptom or duration criteria for a MDE. BPII is distinguished from cyclothymic disorder by the presence of one or more MDEs. *Psychotic disorders, schizophrenia, schizoaffective, and delusional disorder* are all characterized by periods of psychotic symptoms that occur in the absence of prominent mood symptoms. Consider accompanying symptoms, previous course, and family history when differentiating BPII from psychotic disorders.

SOURCE: Adapted from DSM-IV-TR, pp. 392–97.

TABLE 9-11 **CYCLOTHYMIC DISORDERS**

Prevalence and familial pattern	Lifetime prevalence in community is 0.4–1%. Prevalence in mood disorders clinics is 3–5%. MDD, BPI, and BPII appear to be more common among the first-degree relatives of persons with cyclothymic disorder than among the general population. May be an increased familial risk of substance-related disorders and may be more common in the first-degree biological relatives of individuals with BPI.
Core symptoms	The essential feature is a chronic, fluctuating mood disturbance involving numerous periods of hypomanic symptoms and numerous periods of depressive symptoms. The hypomanic symptoms are of insufficient number, severity, pervasiveness, or duration to meet full criteria for a manic episode and the depressive symptoms are of insufficient number, severity, pervasiveness, or duration to meet full criteria for a MDE.
Associated symptoms and disorders	Substance-related disorder and sleep disorders may be present.
Course	Usually begins in adolescence or early adult life. Usually has an insidious onset and chronic course. 15–50% risk that the person will subsequently develop BPI or BPII. Equally common in women and men.
Differential diagnosis	GMC onset late in adult life suggests *Mood Disorder due to a GMC* such as MS. *Substance-induced. BPI disorder with rapid cycling; BPII with rapid cycling*: Both may resemble cyclothymic disorder by virtue of the frequent marked shifts in mood. But by definition the mood states of cyclothymic disorder do not meet the full criteria for a MDE or manic or mixed episode. BPD is associated with marked shifts in mood that may suggest *cyclothymic disorder*. If criteria are met for both, both may be diagnosed.

SOURCE: Adapted from DSM-IV-TR, pp. 398–400.

TABLE 9-12   BIPOLAR NOS

This category includes disorders with bipolar features that do not meet criteria for any specific bipolar disorder.

I.e., very rapid alteration over days between manic and depressive symptoms that do not meet minimal duration criteria for a manic episode or MDE.

I.e., recurrent hypomanic episodes without intercurrent depressive symptoms.

A manic or mixed episode superimposed on delusional disorder, residual schizophrenia, or psychotic disorder NOS.

I.e., hypomanic episodes, along with chronic depressive symptoms, that are too infrequent to qualify for a diagnosis of cyclothymic disorder.

Situations in which the clinician has concluded that a bipolar disorder is present but is unable to determine whether it is primary, due to a GMC, or substance-induced.

SOURCE: Adapted from DSM-IV-TR, pp. 400–401.

TABLE 9-13   BIOPSYCHOSOCIAL TREATMENT OF MOOD DISORDERS

	Bio	Psycho	Social
Major depressive disorder Atypical Melancholic Postpartum	Antidepressants: TCA SSRI Atypical MAOI (see Chapter 3, "Biological Treatment Principles," for dosage information) ECT Light therapy	Individual therapy	Support groups Case management
Dysthymic disorder	Same as above		
Depressive disorder NOS	Same as above		
Bipolar disorders	Mood stabilizers Antipsychotics		

ANXIETY DISORDERS

Anxiety disorders include the following (Tables 9-14 to 9-25):

- Panic disorder
- Panic disorder with agoraphobia
- Panic disorder without agoraphobia
- GAD
- Social phobia
- Simple phobias
- Subtypes, including environmental
- Animal
- Situational
- OCD
- PTSD
- Anxiety disorder NOS

Panic disorder is characterized by recurrent panic attacks. Panic attacks experienced for a month or more alter the individual's behavior (e.g., he becomes more isolated and less engaged in typical activities he previously enjoyed). Symptoms of panic include:

- Pain, numbness, tingling, paresthisias
- Sensation of choking
- Feeling that one is imminently going to die or collapse
- Increased heart rate
- Difficulty breathing
- Sensation of smothering

This event typically crescendos and lasts 10 minutes. It is an excruciating 10 minutes however. It is not unusual for such individuals to present repeatedly to EDs thinking that they are having a heart attack.

Once medical etiologies have been ruled out, the individual may then be referred to the PES/CRC or to a mental health clinician for further care.

The role of the clinician in an emergency setting includes education. A clinician can show empathy by demonstrating knowledge and understanding of the patient's condition and reassuring the patient that the condition is treatable and manageable; explaining the condition in laymen's terms will be helpful.

A survey of what patients want from their doctor revealed that patients want a doctor who is competent and will answer their questions. It is important, particularly in the fast-paced, demanding emergency setting, to be and do both.

Neither panic attacks nor agoraphobia is a codable disorder in the DSM-IV-TR. Both are coded with the specific diagnoses in which they occur.

Panic attack: a discrete period in which there is the sudden onset of intense apprehension, fearfulness, or terror, often associated with feelings of impending doom. During these attacks, symptoms such as shortness of breath, palpitations, chest pain or discomfort, choking or smothering sensations, and fear of "going crazy" or losing control are present. There are three types of panic attacks: (1) unexpected (spontaneous, uncued, out of the blue), (2) situationally bound, and (3) situationally predisposed.

Agoraphobia: anxiety or fear about losing control in public or in a situation in which one is embarrassed or humiliated or in which help is not readily available in the event of having a panic attack or panic like symptoms. Literally *agoraphobia* means "fear of the marketplace."

The biopsychosocial treatment of anxiety disorders is outlined in Table 9-26.

Ideally the emergency clinician should know the community and what services are offered, the quality of those community services, and even individuals at each agency who can be contacted if there is difficulty getting through or making a timely referral. If you have someone you think needs immediate service, it is appropriate to make a specific call to a clinician, if necessary, to set up a timely appointment.

Age and cultural considerations in anxiety disorders are outlined in Tables 9-27 and 9-28.

TABLE 9-14 PANIC DISORDER WITH AGORAPHOBIA

Prevalence and familial pattern	First-degree biological relatives of individuals with PD are up to 8 times more likely to develop PD. If the age of onset of the PD is before 20, first-degree relatives have been found to be up to 20 times more likely to have PD. However, in clinical settings, as many as one-half to three-quarters of individuals with PD do not have an affected first-degree biological relative.
Core symptoms	Recurrent, unexpected panic attacks followed by at least 1 month of persistent concern about having another panic attack, worry about the possible implications or consequences of the panic attacks, or a significant behavioral change related to the attacks; not due to the physiological effects of a substance or a GMC and agoraphobia.
Associated symptoms	In addition to worry about panic attacks and their implications, many also report intermittent or constant feelings of anxiety that are not focused on any specific situation or event. Demoralization is common, attributing this problem to a lack of strength. It may generalize to school, occupational, and interpersonal problems. 10–65% comorbid MDD. In one-third of individuals with both, the depression precedes the onset of PD. In the remaining two-thirds the depression occurs coincident with or following the onset of PD. Substance-related disorders may also occur in a subset of patients trying to treat their anxiety with alcohol or other medications.
Course	Age of onset most typically between late adolescence and the mid-30s. Chronic, waxing-and-waning course. With limited symptoms, attacks experienced with greater frequency if the course of the PD is chronic. Course of agoraphobia and its relationship to the course of panic attacks are variable. Naturalistic follow-up studies of individuals treated in tertiary-care settings suggest that, at 6–10 years post treatment, about 30% of individuals are well, 40–50% are improved but symptomatic, 20–30% the same or worse.
Differential diagnosis	*GMC and substance-induced GMCs* that can cause panic attacks include hyperthyroidism, hyperparathyroidism, pheochromocytoma, vestibular dysfunctions, seizure disorders, and cardiac conditions. CNS stimulants such as amphetamines, caffeine, and cocaine or withdrawal from CNS depressants such as barbiturates and sedative-hypnotics can precipitate panic. Features such as onset after age 45 or the presence of atypical symptoms during a panic attack (e.g., vertigo, loss of consciousness, loss of bladder or bowel control, headaches, and slurred speech) or amnesia suggest a GMC or substance may be causing *anxiety disorders and psychotic disorders*. The presence of unexpected recurrent panic attacks is required for the diagnosis of PD. Panic attacks that occur in the contest of other anxiety disorders are situationally bound stimuli recalling the stressor.

SOURCE: Adapted from DSM-IV-TR, pp. 429–41.

TABLE 9-15 PANIC DISORDER WITH OR WITHOUT AGORAPHOBIA

Prevalence and familial pattern	Lifetime prevalence rates with or without agoraphobia are 1–2% in the community. Of these, one-third to one-half have agoraphobia. In clinical samples 10% of individuals referred for mental health consultation have PD. In general medical settings 10–30%; 60% in cardiology clinics.
Core symptoms	As above with PD.
Associated symptoms	Comorbidity with other anxiety disorders is common. Social phobia and GAD in 15–30% of individuals with PD, specific phobia in 2–20%, and OCD in 10%. PTSD is 2–10%. SAD and hypochondriasis symptoms may also co-occur with PD.
Course	Most typical onset between late adolescence and early 30s Chronic, waxing and waning course.
Differential diagnosis	*PTSD* is cued by, for example, stimuli recalling the stressor. *OCD* is caused by thoughts of or exposure to an object or situation related to an obsession. *GAD* is caused by *social phobia* cued by social situations. *Specific phobia* is caused by a specific feared object or situation. Focus of anxiety helps to differentiate PD with agoraphobia from other disorders characterized by avoidant behaviors. Agoraphobic avoidance is associated with anxiety about the possibility of having a panic attack or panic-like sensations, whereas avoidance in other disorders is associated with concern about the negative or harmful consequences arising from the feared object or situation (e.g., scrutiny, humiliation, and embarrassment in social phobia; falling from a high place in specific phobia of heights; separation from parents in SAD; persecution in delusional disorder). The differential diagnosis of specific phobia, situational type from PD with agoraphobia may be particularly difficult because both disorders may include panic attacks and avoidance of similar types of situations (e.g., driving, flying, public transportation, enclosed places). Four factors helpful in distinguishing between the two disorders: 1. focus of fear 2. type and number of panic attacks 3. number of situations avoided 4. level of intercurrent anxiety Distinguishing between social phobia and PD with agoraphobia can be difficult since both involve panic attacks and avoidance of social situations. The focus of anxiety and the type of panic attacks can help with the distinction. An individual with no prior history of fear of public-speaking experiences a panic attack while giving a talk. If the individual subsequently has panic attacks only in social performance situations and if these attacks are accompanied by a fear of being embarrassed and humiliated, the diagnosis is likely social phobia. But if the attacks become unexpected and occur in other

(continued)

TABLE 9-15   PANIC DISORDER WITH OR WITHOUT AGORAPHOBIA—Continued

situations, then a diagnosis of PD with agoraphobia may be warranted. Individuals with social phobia fear scrutiny and rarely have a panic attack when alone unless anticipating a social situation. An individual with PD with agoraphobia becomes more anxious in situations where he/she must be without a trusted companion.

Nocturnal panic attacks are characteristic of PD.

Sometimes criteria for PD and another anxiety or mood disorder are met and, if so, both disorders should be diagnosed.

SOURCE: Adapted from DSM-IV-TR, pp. 440–43.

TABLE 9-16   **AGORAPHOBIA WITHOUT HISTORY OF PD**

Prevalence and familial predisposition	Unknown.
Core symptoms	Essential features are similar to those of PD with agoraphobia except that the focus of fear is on the occurrence of incapacitation or extremely embarrassing panic-like symptoms or limited-symptom attacks rather than full panic attacks. Full criteria for PD must never have been met.
Associated symptoms	No specific symptoms.
Course	Anecdotal evidence suggests that some cases may persist for years and be associated with considerable impairment.
Differential diagnosis	*PD*, by the absence of a history of recurrent unexpected panic attacks. The individual with *social phobia* avoids social or performance situations in which he/she fears that he/she might act in a way that is humiliating or embarrassing.
	The individual with *specific phobia* avoids a specific feared object or situation.
	The individual with *MDD* may avoid leaving home due to apathy, loss of energy, and anhedonia. Persecutory fears, as in *delusional disorder*, and fears of contamination, as in *OCD*, may lead to widespread avoidance.
	Children with *SAD* avoid situations that take them away from home or close relatives.
	Individuals with *certain GMCs* may avoid situations due to realistic concerns about being incapacitated or being embarassed. The diagnosis of agoraphobia without history of PD should be given only if the fear or avoidance is clearly in excess of that usually associated with the GMC.

SOURCE: Adapted from DSM-IV-TR, pp. 441–43.

TABLE 9-17 SPECIFIC PHOBIA

Prevalence and familial pattern	7.2–11.3% lifetime prevalence rate. There is an increased risk for specific phobias in family members of those with specific phobias. First-degree biological relatives of persons with specific phobias, animal type are likely to have animal phobias, although not necessarily of the same animal.
Core symptoms	Clinically significant anxiety provoked by exposure to a specific feared object or situation often leading to avoidance behavior: • Animal type • Natural environment type • Blood-injection-injury type • Situational type • Other type
Associated symptoms	Restricted lifestyle. Interference with certain occupations. Co-occur with other anxiety disorders, mood disorders, and substance-related disorders, ranging from 50–80% in community samples. In clinical settings, rarely are they the focus of clinical attention; rather they are common comorbid diagnoses with other disorders for which the patient is seeking attention.
Course	Usually first symptoms begin in childhood or early adolescence. Mean age of onset varies according to the type of specific phobia; i.e., situational type tends to be bimodally distributed with a peak in childhood and second peak in the mid-20s; natural environment type, blood-injection-injury type, and animal type usually begin in childhood. Feared objects or situations tend to involve things that may actually represent a threat or have represented a threat at some point in the course of human evolution. Predisposing factors to the onset of specific phobias may include: Traumatic events such as being attacked by an animal or trapped in a closet. Unexpected panic attacks in the to-be-feared situation, observation of others undergoing trauma or demonstrating fearfulness, informational transmission, e.g., repeated parental warnings about the dangers of certain animals. If phobias persist into adulthood, only 20% will remit.
Differential diagnosis	Differ from most other anxiety disorders in levels of intercurrent anxiety; e.g., unlike *panic disorder with agoraphobia*, specific phobias do not present with pervasive anxiety because the fear is limited to specific, circumscribed objects or situations. Differentiating specific phobia, situational type from *PD with agoraphobia* may be particularly difficult because both disorders may include panic attacks and avoidance of similar types of

(continued)

TABLE 9-17   **SPECIFIC PHOBIA—Continued**

situations, e.g., driving, flying, public transportation, enclosed places.

Four factors helpful in distinguishing:

1. focus of fear
2. type and number of panic attacks
3. number of situations avoided
4. level of intercurrent anxiety

Specific and *social phobia* can be differentiated on the basis of the focus of the fears, e.g., avoidance of eating in a restaurant may be based on concerns about negative evaluation from others [social phobia] or concerns about choking [specific phobia].

The avoidance of *PTSD* follows a life-threatening stressor and is accompanied by additional features such as reexperiencing the trauma and restricted affect.

In *OCD*, the avoidance is associated with the content of the obsession, e.g., dirt, contamination.

Social Anxiety Disorder (SAD) involves exclusive fears of separation from persons to whom the individual is attached.

Hypochondriasis and specific phobia, other type involves avoidance of situations that may lead to contracting an illness and depends on the presence or absence of disease conviction. Individuals with hypochondriasis are preoccupied with fears of having a disease, whereas those with specific phobia fear contracting a disease, but do not believe it is already present.

In *anorexia and bulimia nervosa* the avoidance behavior is exclusively limited to avoidance of food and food-related cues. Individuals with *schizophrenia or another psychotic disorder* may avoid certain activities in response to delusions, but do not recognize that the fear is excessive or unreasonable.

Unless there is significant interference with social, educational, or occupational functioning or marked distress about having the phobia, a diagnosis of specific phobia should not be made.

SOURCE: Adapted from DSM-IV-TR, pp. 443–50.

TABLE 9-18 **SOCIAL PHOBIA**

Prevalence and familial pattern	Lifetime prevalence ranges from 3 to 13%. Appears to occur more frequently among first-degree biological relatives.
Core symptoms	Clinically significant anxiety provoked by exposure to certain types of social or performance situations, often leading to avoidance behavior.
Associated symptoms	Hypersensitivity to criticism. Negative evaluation.
Course	Typically has an onset in mid-teens, sometimes emerging out of a childhood history of social inhibition or shyness. Insidious or abrupt following a stressful or humiliating experience. Frequently lifelong, but may attenuate in severity or remit in adulthood.
Differential diagnosis	*Panic Disorder (PD) with agoraphobia and agoraphobia without history of PD*: The situations avoided in social phobia are limited to those involving possible scrutiny by other people. Fears in agoraphobia without PD involve characteristic clusters of situations that may or may not involve scrutiny by others. Also individuals with agoraphobia prefer to be with a trusted companion when in the feared situation, whereas individuals with social phobias may have marked anticipatory anxiety but characteristically do not have a panic attack when alone.
	Persons with *SAD* are usually comfortable in their own home. Those with social phobia may display signs of discomfort when feared social situations occur at home.
	GAD or specific phobia: Neither is the main focus of the individual's anxiety or the fear of embarrassment or humiliation.
	In schizoid personality disorder, social situations are avoided because of lack of interest in relation to other individuals, while individuals with social phobia have a capacity for and interest in social relationships with familiar people.
	Avoidant personality disorder overlaps: Social anxiety may be associated with many other mental disorders and if the symptoms are better accounted for by that disorder, the additional diagnosis of social phobia is not made.
	If social anxiety and avoidance are limited to concerns about a *GMC* such as stuttering, obesity, facial scarring, then the diagnosis of social phobia is not made.
	Finally, performance anxiety, stage fright, and shyness are common and should not be diagnosed as social phobia unless the anxiety or avoidance leads to clinically significant impairment or marked distress.

SOURCE: Adapted from DSM-IV-TR, pp. 450–56.

TABLE 9-19 OBSESSIVE-COMPULSIVE DISORDER

Prevalence and familial pattern	Lifetime prevalence is 2.5% in community samples. Familial pattern: Concordance rate of OCD is higher for monozygotic twins than it is for dizygotic twins.
Core symptoms	Obsessions that cause marked anxiety or distress and/or compulsions that serve to neutralize anxiety.
Associated symptoms	High incidence of OCD in children and adults with Tourette's syndrome—35–50%. Incidence of Tourette's in OCD is 5–7%. In adults, OCD may be associated with MDD, other anxiety disorders, eating disorders, and personality disorders (e.g., OCPD, avoidant personality disorder, dependent personality disorder). In children, it may be associated with learning disorders and disruptive behavior disorders.
Course	Modal age of onset is earlier in males than females; between ages 6 and 15 years for males, 20 and 29 for females. Typically onset is gradual. Majority have a chronic waxing-and-waning course, with exacerbation of symptoms that may be related to stress. 15% show progressive deterioration in occupational and social functioning. 5% have an episodic course with minimal or no symptoms between episodes.
Differential diagnosis	*Anxiety disorder due to a GMC.* *Substance-induced anxiety.* *Body dysmorphic disorder*—preoccupation with appearance. *Specific or social phobia*—preoccupation with a feared object or situation. *Trichotillomania—hair pulling.* *MDE:* a depressed individual who ruminates that he is worthless would not be considered to have obsessions because such brooding is not egodystonic. *GAD*, which is characterized by excessive worry distinct from obsessions since the worry is about real-life circumstances. *Hypochondriasis*—fears of having, or the idea that one has, a serious disease based on misinterpretation of bodily symptoms. If the concern is about rituals such as accompany having an illness or excessive washing or checking behavior related to concerns about the illness or about spreading it to other people, an additional *OCD* diagnosis may be warranted. If the major concern is about contacting an illness rather than having an illness and no rituals are involved, *specific phobia* may be appropriate. In some individuals with OCD, reality testing is lost and the obsession may reach delusional proportions thus warranting an additionally diagnosis of *delusional disorder or psychotic disorder NOS*. The specifier "with *poor insight*" may be useful for those on the boundary between obsession and delusion.

(continued)

TABLE 9-19   OBSESSIVE-COMPULSIVE DISORDER—Continued

Schizophrenia: ruminative delusional thoughts and bizarre, stereotyped behaviors. In schizophrenia these are not ego-dystonic and not subject to reality testing. Occasionally both may occur.

Tics and stereotyped movements must be distinguished from compulsions.

A *tic* is a sudden, rapid, recurrent, nonrhythmic stereotyped motor movement or vocalization (e.g., eye blinking, tongue protrusion, throat clearing).

Stereotyped movement is a repetitive, seemingly driven nonfunctional motor behavior (e.g., head banging, body rocking, self-biting). In contrast to compulsions, tics and stereotyped movements are typically less complex and are not aimed at neutralizing an obsession. They may coexist.

Activities such as eating *(eating disorders)*, sexual behaviors (*paraphilias*), gambling (e.g., *pathological gambling),* or substance use (*alcohol dependence or abuse*), when engaged in excessively, are sometimes called compulsive. This is a misnomer in that the person usually derives pleasure from the activity and may wish to resist it only because of its negative consequences.

OCPD is not characterized by the presence of obsessions or compulsions and instead involves a pervasive pattern of preoccupation with orderliness, perfectionism, and control.

SOURCE: Adapted from DSM-IV-TR, pp. 456–63.

TABLE 9-20 POSTTRAUMATIC STRESS DISORDER

Prevalence and familial pattern	Lifetime prevalence of 8% of the adult population in the United States. There is evidence of a heritable component to the transmission of PTSD. Also, a history of depression in first-degree biological relatives has been related to an increased vulnerability to developing PTSD.
Core symptoms	Reexperiencing of an extremely traumatic event accompanied by symptoms of increased arousal and by avoidance of stimuli associated with the trauma.
Associated symptoms	• Survival guilt is common • Avoidance patterns • In severe cases auditory hallucinations and paranoid ideation • Symptoms seen in those with an interpersonal stressor, e.g., childhood sexual or physical abuse, domestic battering • Impaired affect modulation • Self-destructive and impulsive behavior • Dissociative symptoms • Somatic complaints • Feelings of ineffectiveness, shame, despair, or hopelessness • Feeling permanently damaged • A loss of previously sustained beliefs • Hostility • Social withdrawal • Feeling constantly threatened, impaired relationships with others • Change in the individual's previous personality characteristics
Course	Can occur at any age. Symptoms usually begin within the first 3 months after the trauma although there may be a delay of months or even years. Symptoms and relative predominance of experiencing, avoidance, and hyperarousal symptoms may vary over time. Duration of symptoms varies, complete recovery occurring within 3 months in approximately half the cases. Symptom reactivation may occur in response to reminders of the original trauma, life stressors, or new traumatic events. Severity, duration, and proximity of an individual's exposure to the traumatic event are the most important factors affecting the likelihood of developing this disorder. Social supports, family history, childhood experiences, personality variables, and preexisting mental disorders may influence the development of PTSD. If the stressor is extreme, individuals can develop PTSD symptoms without any predisposing conditions.
Differential diagnosis	*Adjustment disorder*—The stressor can be of any severity. Symptoms of avoidance, numbing, and increased arousal that are present before exposure to the stressor do not meet criteria for PTSD.

(continued)

TABLE 9-20   **POSTTRAUMATIC STRESS DISORDER—Continued**

If the symptoms response pattern to the extreme stressor meets criteria for another mental disorder, (e.g., *brief psychotic disorder, MDD*), these diagnoses may be given instead of or in addition to PTSD.

Differentiate *acute stress disorder (ASD)* from PTSD because the symptom pattern in ASD must occur within 4 weeks of the traumatic event and resolve within that 4-week period. If the symptoms persist longer than 1 month than the diagnosis is changed from ASD to PTSD.

OCD—There are recurrent intrusive thoughts, but these are experienced as inappropriate and are not related to an experience traumatic event.

Differentiate flashbacks in PTSD from hallucinations and other perceptual disturbances that may occur in *schizophrenia, other psychotic disorders, mood disorders with psychotic features, a delirium, substance-induced disorders, and psychotic disorders due to a GMC.*

Malingering should also be ruled out in those situations in which financial remuneration, benefit eligibility, and forensic determinations play a role.

SOURCE: Adapted from DSM-IV-TR, pp. 463–68.

TABLE 9-21 ACUTE STRESS DISORDER

Prevalence and familial pattern	Prevalence in the general population is not known.
Core symptoms	Symptoms similar to those of PTSD that occur immediately in the aftermath of an extremely traumatic event.
Associated symptoms and conditions	Despair and hopelessness; MDD may develop. Survivor guilt. Increased risk to develop PTSD.
Course	Symptoms are experienced during or immediately after the trauma, last for at least 2 days, and either resolve within 4 weeks after the conclusion of the traumatic event or the diagnosis is changed (i.e., if the symptoms last longer than 1 month, the disorder is PTSD). The most important factors in determining the likelihood of development of ASD are severity, duration, and proximity of an individual's exposure to the traumatic event. Social supports, family history, childhood experiences, personality variables, and preexisting mental disorders may influence the development of PTSD. If the stressor is extreme, individuals can develop ASD without any predisposing conditions.
Differential diagnosis	*Mental disorder due to a GMC and a substance-induced disorder brief psychotic disorder* in those experiencing psychotic symptoms following an extreme stressor. *MDD.* *An exacerbation of a preexisting mental disorder.* *PTSD*—duration. *Adjustment disorder* for those individuals who have an extreme stressor but who develop a symptom pattern that does not meet criteria for ASD. *Malingering.* *Delirium*—a separate diagnosis of anxiety disorder due to a GMC is not given if the anxiety disturbance occurs exclusively during the course of a delirium. *Dementia*—anxiety disorder due to a GMC can co-occur with dementia if the anxiety is a direct etiological consequence of the pathological process causing the dementia and is a prominent part of the clinical presentation. *Substance-induced anxiety disorder.* *Primary anxiety disorder.* *Adjustment disorder with anxiety or with mixed anxiety and depressed mood* (e.g., a maladaptive response to the stress of having a GMC). Late age of onset and the absence of a personal or family history of anxiety disorders suggest the need for a through assessment to rule out the diagnosis of *anxiety disorder due to a GMC. Anxiety NOS* is diagnosed if the clinician cannot determine whether the anxiety disturbance is primary, substance-induced, or due to a general medical condition.

SOURCE: Adapted from DSM-IV-TR, pp. 469–72.

TABLE 9-22 GENERALIZED ANXIETY DISORDER (GAD)

Prevalence and familial pattern	Lifetime prevalence is 5% in community sample. In anxiety disorder clinics, up to a quarter of the individuals have GAD.
Core symptoms	At least 6 months of persistent and excessive anxiety and worry more days than not about a number of events or activities.
Associated symptoms and conditions	Co-occurs with mood disorders. Other anxiety disorders. Substance-related disorders. Conditions associated with stress (e.g., IBS, headaches) may frequently accompany GAD.
Course	Anxiety occurs in response to a life stressor and does not persist for more than 6 months after the termination of the stressor or its consequences.
Differential diagnosis	Generalized anxiety is common during *mood and psychotic disorders* but should not be diagnosed separately if it occurs exclusively during the course of these conditions. *Nonpathological anxiety.* Worries with GAD are difficult to control and typically interfere significantly with functioning. Worries of everyday life are perceived as more controllable and can be put off until later. Worries associated with GAD are more pervasive, pronounced, distressing, and have longer duration and frequently occur without precipitants. The more life circumstances about which the person worries excessively (finances, children's safety, job performance, car repairs), the more likely the diagnosis. Everyday worries are much less likely to be accompanied by physical symptoms (e.g., excessive fatigue, restlessness, feeling keyed up or on edge, irritability).
Core symptoms	Disorders with prominent anxiety or phobic avoidance that do not meet criteria for any of the specific anxiety disorders or anxiety symptoms about which there is inadequate or contradictory information. Examples: Mixed anxiety-depressive disorder: clinically significant symptoms of anxiety and depression but the criteria are not met for either a specific mood disorder or a specific anxiety disorder. Clinically significant social phobic symptoms that are related to the social impact of having a GMC or mental disorder (e.g., Parkinson's disease, dermatological conditions, stuttering, anorexia nervosas, body dysmorphic disorder). Situations in which the disturbance is severe enough to warrant a diagnosis of an anxiety disorder but the individual fails to report enough symptoms for the full criteria of any specific anxiety disorder to have been met. Situations in which the clinician has concluded that an anxiety disorder is present but is unable to determine whether it is primary, due to a general medical condition, or substance-induced.

SOURCE: Adapted from DSM-IV-TR, pp. 472–76.

TABLE 9-23 **ANXIETY DISORDER NOS**

Core symptoms	Prominent Anxiety or phobic avoidance that does not meet criteria for any specific anxiety disorder or adjustment disorder. Mixed anxiety and depressed mood. Examples include:

1. Mixed anxiety—depressed.
2. Clinically significant social phobic symptoms that are related to the social impact of having a GMC or mental disorder.
3. Situations in which the disturbance is severe enough to warrant a diagnosis of an anxiety disorder, but doesn't meet full criteria for any specific anxiety disorder.
4. Clinician has concluded an anxiety disorder is present but is unable to determine whether it is primary, due to a general medical condition, or substance-induced.

Source: Adapted from DSM-IV-TR, p. 484.

TABLE 9-24 **ANXIETY DISORDER DUE TO A GMC**

Core symptoms	Prominent symptoms of anxiety that are judged to be a direct physiological consequence of a GMC

Specifiers:

   With generalized anxiety
   With panic attacks
   With obsessive-compulsive symptoms
   With phobic symptoms
   Endocrine conditions
   Cardiovascular conditions
   Respiratory conditions
   Metabolic
   Neurological conditions

Source: Adapted from DSM-IV-TR, pp. 476–79.

TABLE 9-25 **SUBSTANCE-INDUCED ANXIETY DISORDER**

Prevalence and familial pattern	Unknown.
Core symptoms	Prominent symptoms of anxiety that are judged to be a direct physiological consequence of a drug of abuse, a medication, or toxin exposure. Specifiers: With generalized anxiety With panic attacks With obsessive-compulsive symptoms With phobic symptoms With onset during intoxication With onset during withdrawal
Differential diagnosis	Anxiety symptoms commonly occur in substance intoxication and substance withdrawal. The diagnosis of the substance-specific intoxication or substance-specific withdrawal usually suffices to categorize. Only when the anxiety symptoms are judged to be in excess of those usually associated with the intoxication or withdrawal syndrome and when the anxiety symptoms are sufficiently severe to warrant independent clinical attention should the diagnosis of substance-induced anxiety disorder be made. If substance-induced anxiety symptoms occur exclusively during the course of a delirium, the anxiety symptoms are considered to be an associated feature of the delirium and are not diagnosed separately. Rule out a primary anxiety disorder. A substance-induced anxiety disorder due to a prescribed treatment for a mental disorder or GMC must have its onset while the person is receiving the medication or during withdrawal, if a withdrawal syndrome is associated with the medication. Once the treatment is discontinued, the anxiety symptoms will usually improve markedly or remit within days to several weeks to a month (depending on the half-life of the substance and the presence of a withdrawal syndrome). If symptoms persist beyond 4 weeks, other causes for the anxiety symptoms should be considered. Rule out GMC. When there is insufficient evidence to determine whether the anxiety symptoms are due to a substance, including a medication, or to a general medical condition or are primary, anxiety disorder NOS is indicated.

SOURCE: Adapted from DSM-IV-TR, pp. 479–83.

TABLE 9-26   **BIOPSYCHOSOCIAL TREATMENT OF ANXIETY DISORDERS**

	Biological	Psychological	Social
Panic disorder with agoraphobia	SSRI Short-term BZ	CBT Desensitization In vitro, in vivo Flooding	Group therapy Supportive, CBT, process
Panic disorder without agoraphobia	SSRI Short-term BZ		
Social phobia	SSRI Propanolol	CBT Exposure	Group CBT Groups like Toastmasters
Simple phobias		CBT Systematic desensitization	Group

PTSD	SSRI	Life review
		Individual therapy
		    that helps the
		    individual to
		    review the
		    traumatic events,
		    process them, and
		    integrate and move
		    on in life
			Support pro-
			    cess–oriented
			    group where
			    people with a
			    shared trau-
			    matic experi-
			    ence can share
			    their experi-
			    ences

OCD	SSRI Clomipramine	CBT Exposure	Support You Are Not Alone

TABLE 9-27   **AGE CONSIDERATIONS**

	Children/Adolescents
Panic disorder	Age of onset typically between late adolescence and mid-30s.
Agoraphobia	Rarely associated with childhood onset.
Specific phobia	Children may express by crying, tantrums, freezing, or clinging. They often do not recognize that their fears are excessive or unreasonable and rarely report. Only if the fears lead to clinically significant impairment should the diagnosis be given.
	The Elderly
	No specific concerns related to age.

Source: Adapted from DSM-IV-TR, pp. 429–84.

TABLE 9-28 CULTURAL CONSIDERATIONS

Panic disorder	In some cultures, panic attacks may involve intense fear of witchcraft or magic.
Agoraphobia	Some cultures restrict the participation of women in public life; this must be distinguished from agoraphobia.
Specific phobia	Fears of magic or spirits are present in many cultures; only if the fear is excessive in the context of that culture and causes significant impairment or distress should it be diagnosed.

SOURCE: Adapted from DSM-IV-TR, pp. 429–84.

BIBLIOGRAPHY

Diagnostic and Statistical Manual of Mental Disorders, 4th ed., Text Revision (DSM-IV-TR). Washington, DC: American Psychological Association, 2000.

Medication Treatment of Bipolar Disorder. A Postgraduate Medicine Special Report. Postgraduate Medicine, 2000.

Quick Reference to the American Psychiatric Association Practice Guidelines for the Treatment of Psychiatric Disorders: Compendium 2000. Arlington, VA: American Psychiatric Association, 2002.

Young S, et al. Depression in Women of Reproductive Age. *Postgraduate Medicine* 112(3) (2002).

Chapter 10

SUBSTANCE USE DISORDERS

INTRODUCTION

In 1999, an estimated 14.8 million Americans used illicit drugs. That same year, 3.6 million Americans met diagnostic criteria for dependence on illicit drugs. That same year, 3.6 million Americans met diagnostic criteria for dependence on illicit drugs; 1.1 million were age 12–17. The Epidemiologic Catchment Area (ECA) studies estimate that 13.8% of Americans will have an alcohol-related substance abuse disorder (SUD) in their life, and 30–55% of those with mental illness also have a comorbid SUD. A total of 100,000 deaths per year are alcohol-related. The suicide rate is 5–6% among those with alcohol dependence. Twenty-five percent of general hospital admissions involve patients with problems related to chronic alcohol use, such as cirrhosis, or cardiomyopathy, or related to withdrawal, e.g., seizures, pneumonia, liver failure, and subdural hematomas.

The goals of this chapter include:

1. Review DSM-IV-TR criteria for substance abuse, substance dependence, substance intoxication, and substance withdrawal
2. Review general guidelines of emergency assessment and treatment of substance use disorders

3. Review DSM-IV-TR criteria for selected substance use disorders including culture/age/gender
4. Review biopsychosocial emergency assessment and management of selected substance use disorders

REVIEW OF CLASSIFICATION OF SUBSTANCE USE DISORDERS

The substance-related disorders are divided into two groups:

1. Substance use disorders
   - Substance dependence
   - Substance abuse
2. Substance-induced disorders
   - Substance intoxication
   - Substance withdrawal
   - Substance-induced delirium
   - Substance-induced persisting dementia
   - Substance-induced persisting amnestic disorder
   - Substance-induced psychotic amnestic disorder
   - Substance-induced mood disorder
   - Substance-induced anxiety disorder
   - Substance-induced sexual dysfunction
   - Substance-induced sleep disorder

There are 13 classes of substances. They are:

- Alcohol
- Amphetamine
- Cocaine
- Cannabis
- Caffeine
- Hallucinogens
- Inhalants
- Nicotine
- Opioids
- Phencyclidine
- Sedative hypnotics
- Other
- Polysubstance

REVIEW OF DSM-IV-TR CRITERIA (TABLE 10-1)

There is prolonged heavy use of the substance. In this state, the person will likely take the substance to relieve or to avoid unpleasant withdrawal symptoms.

According to DSM-IV-TR, dependence can be noted as mild, moderate, or severe and remission may be noted to be partial or early (Tables 10-2 through 10-5).

COURSE AND REMISSION SPECIFIERS FOR SUBSTANCE DEPENDENCE

- With or without physiological dependence (tolerance or withdrawal)
- Remission subtypes include full, early partial, sustained, and sustained partial
- Remission—on agonist or for those living in a controlled drug-free environment

TABLE 10-1   DSM-IV-TR CRITERIA FOR SUBSTANCE DEPENDENCE

A maladaptive pattern of substance use, leading to clinically significant impairment or distress, as manifested by three or more of the following, occurring at any time in the same 12-month period:

1. Tolerance, as defined by either of the following:
   a. A need for markedly increased amounts of the substance to achieve intoxication or desired effect.
   b. Markedly diminished effect with continued use of the same amount of the substance.
2. Withdrawal, as manifested by either of the following:
   a. The characteristic withdrawal syndrome for the substance (refer to Criteria a and b of the criteria sets for withdrawal from the specific substances).
   b. The same (or a closely related) substance is taken to relieve or avoid withdrawal symptoms.
3. The substance is often taken in larger amounts or over a longer period than was intended.
4. There is a persistent desire or unsuccessful efforts to cut down or control substance use.
5. A great deal of time is spent in activities necessary to obtain the substance (e.g., visiting multiple doctors or driving long distances), use the substance (e.g., chain smoking), or recover from its effects.
6. Important social, occupational, or recreational activities are given up or reduced because of substance use.
7. The substance use is continued despite knowledge of having a persistent or recurrent physical or psychological problem that is likely to have been caused or exacerbated by the substance (e.g., current cocaine use despite recognition of cocaine-induced depression, or continued drinking despite recognition that an ulcer was made worse by alcohol consumption).

SOURCE: Adapted from DSM-IV-TR, pp. 197–98.

TABLE 10-2 DSM-IV-TR CRITERIA FOR SUBSTANCE ABUSE

A. A maladaptive pattern of substance use leading to clinically significant impairment or distress, as manifested by one or more of the following occurring within a 12-month period:

   (1) Recurrent substance use resulting in a failure to fulfill major role obligations at work, school, or home (e.g., repeated absences or poor work performance related to substance use; substance-related absences, suspensions, or expulsions from school; neglect of children or household).

   (2) Recurrent substance use in situations in which it is physically hazardous (e.g., driving an automobile or operating a machine when impaired by a substance).

   (3) Recurrent substance-related legal problems (e.g., arrests for substance-related disorderly conduct).

   (4) Continued substance use despite having persistent or recurrent social or interpersonal problems caused or exacerbated by the effects of the substance (e.g., arguments with spouse about consequences of intoxication, physical fights).

B. The symptoms have never met the criteria for substance dependence for this class of substance.

Source: Adapted from DSM-IV-TR, pp. 198–99.

TABLE 10-3 DSM-IV-TR CRITERIA FOR SUBSTANCE INTOXICATION

A. The development of a reversible substance-specific syndrome due to recent ingestion or exposure to a substance. Note: Different substances may produce similar or identical syndromes.

B. Clinically significant maladaptive behavioral or psychological changes that are due to the effect of the substance on the central nervous system (e.g., belligerence, mood liability, cognitive impairment, impaired judgment, impaired social or occupational functioning) and develop during or shortly after use of the substance.

C. The symptoms are not due to a general medical condition and are not better accounted for by another mental disorder.

Source: Adapted from DSM-IV-TR, pp. 199–201.

TABLE 10-4 DSM-IV-TR CRITERIA FOR SUBSTANCE WITHDRAWAL

A. The development of a substance-specific syndrome due to the cessation of or reduction in substance use that has been heavy and prolonged.

B. The substance-specific syndrome causes clinically significant distress or impairment in social, occupational, or other important areas of functioning.

C. The symptoms are not due to a general medical condition and are not better accounted for by another mental disorder.

Source: Adapted from DSM-IV-TR, pp. 201–2.

TABLE 10-5   ASSOCIATED FEATURES OF SUBSTANCE DEPENDENCE, ABUSE, INTOXICATION, AND WITHDRAWAL (DSM-IV-TR)

Assessment	Detailed history from the individual and collateral sources. Physical exam and lab test results.
Route of administration	IV, "snorting," and smoking a substance tends to produce a more rapid, efficient absorption into the bloodstream, a more intense intoxication, and increased likelihood of an escalating pattern of substance use leading to dependence since these routes of administration quickly deliver a large amount of the substance to the brain and thus are associated with higher levels of substance consumption and increased likelihood of toxic effects (e.g., IV amphetamine user is more likely to rapidly consume large amounts of the substance and thereby risk an overdose than the PO amphetamine user).
Speed of onset within a class of substance	Rapidly acting substances are more likely than slower-acting substances to produce immediate intoxication and lead to dependence or abuse (e.g., diazepam and alprazolam have a more rapid onset than phenobarbital and thus may consequently be more likely to lead to substance dependence or abuse).
Duration of effects	Relatively short-acting substances (certain anxiolytics) tend to have a higher potential for the development of dependence or abuse than substances with similar effects that have a longer duration. The half-life of the substance parallels aspects of withdrawal: the longer the duration of action, the longer the time between cessation and the onset of withdrawal symptoms and the longer the withdrawal is likely to last (e.g., with heroin, the onset of acute withdrawal symptoms is more rapid but the withdrawal syndrome is less persistent than for methadone. In general, the longer the acute withdrawal period, the less intense the syndrome tends to be.).
Use of multiple substances	Often involve several substances used simultaneously or sequentially (e.g., individuals with cocaine dependence frequently also use anxiolytics or opioids, often to counteract lingering cocaine-induced anxiety symptoms); individuals with opioid dependence or cannabis dependence usually have several other substance-related disorders, most often involving alcohol, anxiolytics, amphetamine, or cocaine.
Associated laboratory findings	Laboratory analyses of blood and urine samples can help to determine the recent use of a substance. A positive blood or urine test, however, does not by itself indicate that the individual has a pattern of substance use that meets the criteria for a substance-related disorder and a negative blood or urine test does not by itself rule out a diagnosis of a substance-related disorder.
	In the case of intoxication, blood and urine tests can help to determine the relevant substances involved. Specific confirmation of the suspected substance may require toxicological analysis, because various substances have similar intoxication syndromes; individuals often take a number of different substances; substitu-

(continued)

	tion and contamination of street drugs is frequent; those who obtain substances illicitly often do not know the specific contents of what they have taken. Toxicological tests may also help in differential diagnosis to determine the role of the substance intoxication or withdrawal in the etiology or exacerbation of symptoms of a variety of mental disorders.
	Serial blood levels may help to differentiate intoxication from withdrawal. Blood concentration of a substance may be a useful clue in determining whether the person has a high tolerance to a given group of substances (e.g., a person presenting with a BAL of over 150 mg/dL without signs of alcohol intoxication has a significant tolerance to alcohol and is likely to be a chronic user of either alcohol or a sedative, hypnotic, or anxiolytic). Determining the individual's response to an agonist medication can also assess tolerance. Evidence for cessation or reduction of dosing may also be obtained by lab tests and history. Although many substances and their metabolites clear the urine within 48 hours of ingestion, certain metabolites may present for a longer period than in those who use the substance chronically. If an individual presents with withdrawal from an unknown substance, urine tests may help identify the substance from which the person is withdrawing and make it possible to initiate appropriate treatment. Urine tests may also be helpful in differentiation of withdrawal from other mental disorders, because withdrawal symptoms can mimic the symptoms of mental disorders unrelated to use of a substance.
Associated physical examination findings and general medical conditions	In general, intoxication with amphetamines or cocaine is accompanied by increases in blood pressure, respiratory rate, pulse, and body temperature. Intoxication with sedative, hypnotic, or antianxiety substances or with opioid medication often involves the opposite pattern. Substance dependence and abuse are often associated with general medication conditions often related to the toxic effects of the substances on particular organ systems (e.g., cirrhosis in alcohol dependence) or the routes of administration (e.g., human immunodeficiency virus [HIV] infection from shared needles).
Associated mental disorders	When mental disorder symptoms are judged to be a direct physiological consequence of a substance, a substance-induced disorder is diagnosed. Substance-related disorders are commonly comorbid with, and complicate the course and treatment of, many mental disorders (e.g., conduct disorder in adolescents, antisocial and borderline personality disorders, schizophrenia, bipolar disorders).
Cultural age and gender features	Patterns of substance use, accessibility of substances, physiological reactions to substances, and prevalence of substance-related disorders vary according to culture age and gender. Black men and women appear at much higher risk for drug-related mortality than

(continued)

	their white counterparts. The evaluation of any individual's pattern of substance use must take these factors into account. Individuals between 18 and 24 have a relatively high prevalence rate for the use of virtually every substance. For drugs of abuse, intoxication is usually the initial substance-related disorder; it usually begins in the teens. Withdrawal can occur at any age as long as the relevant drug has been taken in high enough doses over a long-enough period of time. Dependence can occur at any age, but typically has its initial onset for most drugs of abuse in the 20s, 30s, and 40s. Substance-related disorders are usually diagnosed more commonly in males than females, but the sex ratios vary with class of substance.
Course	Course varies with substance, route of administration, and other factors. Intoxication usually develops within minutes after a sufficiently large single dose and continues or intensifies with frequently repeated doses. The onset of intoxication may be delayed with slowly absorbed substances or with those that must be metabolized to active compounds. Long-acting substances may produce prolonged intoxications. Withdrawal develops with the decline of the substance in the CNS. Early symptoms of withdrawal usually develop a few hours after dosing stops for substances with short elimination half-lives (e.g., alcohol, lorezapam, or heroin).
	Although withdrawal seizures may develop several weeks after termination of high doses of a long-half-life anxiolytic substance, the more intense signs of withdrawal usually end within a few days to a few weeks after the cessation of substance use, although some subtle physiological signs may be detectable for many weeks or even months as part of a protracted withdrawal syndrome, e.g., impaired sleep for months after an alcohol-dependent individual stops drinking.
	Substance abuse is likely to evolve into substance dependence with those substances that have a high potential for the development of tolerance, withdrawal, and patterns of compulsive use such as cocaine and heroin. The course of substance dependence is variable, but typically chronic, lasting years, with periods of exacerbation and partial or full remission. There may be periods of heavy intake and severe problems, periods of total abstinence, and times of nonproblematic use of the substance sometimes lasting for months. Sometimes substance dependence is brief and self-limited, and/or associated with spontaneous, long-term remissions. Follow-ups reveal that 20% or more of individuals with alcohol dependence become permanently abstinent, usually following a severe life stress (e.g., the threat or imposition of social or legal sanctions, discovery of a life-threatening medical condition). The first 12 months after the onset of a remission is a particularly vulnerable time for the individual to relapse. Many

(continued)

	become cavalier about their sobriety and underestimate their vulnerability to redeveloping a pattern of dependence. The presence of co-occurring mental disorders (e.g., ASPD, BPD, untreated MDD, bipolar disorders) often increases the risk of complications and a poor outcome.
Impairment and complications	Malnutrition and GMCs may result from improper diet and inadequate personal hygiene.
	Intoxication or withdrawal may be complicated by trauma related to impaired motor coordination or faulty judgment. Material used to "cut" certain substances can produce toxic or allergic reactions.
	Using substances intranasally, "snorting," may cause erosion of the nasal septum.
	Stimulant use can result in sudden death from cardiac arrhythmia, myocardial infarction, a cerebrovascular accident, or respiratory arrest.
	Contaminated needles during IV use can cause HIV, hepatitis, tetanus, vasculitis, septicemia, subacute bacterial endocarditis, embolic phenomena, and malaria.
	Substance use can be associated with violent or aggressive behavior, fights, and criminal activity and can result in injury to the person using the substance or to others. Approximately one-half of all highway fatalities involve either a driver or a pedestrian who is intoxicated. In addition, approximately 10% of individuals with substance dependence commit suicide, often in the context of a substance-induced mood disorder.
	Finally, because most of the substances cross the placenta, they may have potential adverse effects on the developing fetus (FAE, FAS). When taken repeatedly by the mother, a number of substances (e.g., cocaine, opioids, alcohol, and sedatives, hypnotics, and anxiolytics) are capable of causing physiological dependence in the fetus and a withdrawal syndrome in the newborn.
Familial pattern	Substance abuse and substance dependence may aggregate in families; some of this may be explained by the concurrent familial distribution of ASPD, which may predispose individuals to the development of substance abuse or dependence. Children of individuals with ASPD have a predisposition to developing substance dependence on all substances; children of individuals with alcohol dependence only are at higher risk for developing alcohol dependence.
Differential diagnosis	Nonpathological substance use or social drinking.
	Use of medications for appropriate medical purposes:
	Distinguish by the presence of a pattern of multiple symptoms occurring over an extended period of time (e.g., tolerance, withdrawal, compulsive use) or the presence of substance-related problems (e.g., medical complications, disruption in social and family relationships, vocational or financial difficulties, legal problems).

(continued)

Intoxication: One or more episodes of intoxication alone are not sufficient for a diagnosis of either substance dependence or abuse.

Intoxication vs. withdrawal: Sometimes this is difficult to distinguish. If a symptom arises during the time of dosing and then gradually abates after dosing stops, it is likely to be part of intoxication. If the symptoms arise after stopping the substance or reducing its use, it is likely to be part of withdrawal.

However, individuals with substance-related disorders often take more than one substance and may be intoxicated with one substance (e.g., heroin) while withdrawing from another (e.g., diazepam). This differential is further complicated by the fact the signs and symptoms of withdrawal from some substances (e.g., sedatives) may partially mimic intoxication with others (e.g., amphetamines).

Substance intoxication delirium:

Substance-induced psychotic disorder with onset during intoxication

Substance-induced mood disorder with onset during intoxication

Substance-induced anxiety disorder with onset during intoxication

Substance-induced sexual dysfunction with onset during intoxication

Substance-induced sleep disorder with onset during intoxication

All are differentiated from substance intoxication by the fact the symptoms of these disorders are in excess of those usually associated with substance intoxication and are severe enough to warrant independent clinical attention.

Substance withdrawal delirium:

Substance-induced psychotic disorder with onset during withdrawal

Substance-induced mood disorder with onset during withdrawal

Substance-induced anxiety disorder with onset during withdrawal

Substance-induced sexual dysfunction with onset during withdrawal

Substance-induced sleep disorder with onset during withdrawal

All are distinguished from substance withdrawal by the fact the symptoms in these disorders are in excess of those usually associated with substance withdrawal and are severe enough to warrant independent clinical attention.

Symptoms of preexisting mental disorders exacerbated by substance intoxication or withdrawal: An additional diagnosis of substance-induced disorder is usually not made under these circumstances although a diagnosis of substance intoxication or withdrawal might be appropriate; e.g., intoxication with some substances may exacerbate the mood swings in bipolar disorder, the auditory hallucinations and paranoid delusions in schizophrenia, the intrusive thoughts and terrifying dreams in PTSD, and anxiety symptoms in PD, GAD, social phobia, and agoraphobia. Intoxication

(continued)

or withdrawal may also increase the risk of suicide, violence, and impulsive behavior in individuals with a preexisting antisocial or borderline personality disorder.

Neurological or metabolic conditions: sometimes produce symptoms that resemble and are sometimes misattributed to intoxication or withdrawal (e.g., fluctuating levels of consciousness, slurred speech, incoordination).

Symptoms of infectious diseases may also mimic withdrawal (e.g., viral gastroenteritis can be similar to opioid withdrawal).

Mental disorder due to a general medical condition: This should be diagnosed if the symptoms are judged to be a direct physiological consequence of a GMC. If the symptoms are judged to be a direct physiological consequence of both substance use and a GMC, both a substance-related disorder and a mental disorder due to a GMC may be diagnosed.

NOS category is appropriate if the clinician is unable to determine whether the presenting symptoms are substance-induced, due to a GMC, or primary.

SOURCE: Adapted from DSM-IV-TR, pp. 202–12.

GENERAL MANAGEMENT/APPROACH IN THE EMERGENCY PHASE

Bear in mind the unique goals in the emergency assessment and treatment of all substance use disorders. Psychiatric management of said disorders has a number of objectives. It is wise to consider these as phasic with the emergency phase typically involving the treatment of intoxication/withdrawal. A more detailed assessment phase leading to the development of a comprehensive treatment strategy is the focus of nonemergency phases. This does not mean that the emergency clinician should not know or attend to the importance of these phases. Indeed, patients may have questions about treatment, what to expect, and so on, and the emergency clinician should be prepared to encourage and educate patients on these issues. But the chief aim of all emergency measures is to stabilize as quickly as possible and determine the most appropriate treatment disposition. The following list gives the illusion that management is neatly stepwise when in reality, it is often simultaneous and overlapping (i.e., a nonlinear process).

1. Establish a therapeutic rapport. The emergency clinician is likely to encounter denial and other negative attitudes about treatment. Encouragement and instillation of hope for recovery and a healthy life is particularly important at this stage.
2. Assess substances abused, route of administration, dose, and time of last use. Monitor clinical status and manage intoxication and withdrawal states. There is a complexity to this as signs and symptoms of withdrawal vary according to the substance used, concurrent GMCs or other psychiatric disorders, and concomitant use of other illicit drugs or prescribed medications. The disorder rarely involves a tidy use of just one drug. Many patients use multiple substances to enhance, ameliorate, or modify the degree or nature of their intoxication or to relieve withdrawal symptoms.
3. History, physical exam, and pertinent labs.
4. Collateral information with the patient's permission if possible—friends, spouse, case manager, treating psychiatrist, medical record if available for review.
5. Stomach decontamination (i.e., gastric lavage) or techniques that increase the rate of excretion of drugs or their active metabolites. Or drugs such as naloxone, an opioid antagonist, may be given to antagonize or reverse the effects of the abused substance.
6. Decrease external stimulation, provide orientation and reality testing.
7. Support with medications to ease withdrawal symptoms or other negative effects from the drug use such as induced psychosis or anxiety; psychological-supportive, encouraging, reassuring, calm, respectful, and social: facilitating a family intervention, peer support of AA members, group referral, AA.
8. In this phase of treatment, medications to treat intoxication and withdrawal states and medications to treat comorbid psychiatric conditions are most appropriate. Pharmacotherapies that are directed to decrease the reinforcing defects of an abused substance or discourage the use of substances and agonist substitution therapy are not typically part of this phase of treatment although the clinician should certainly be familiar with these medications.
9. Psychosocial treatments include cognitive-behavioral therapies, group therapies, family therapies, and self-help groups.
10. CD evaluation and referral—inpatient, outpatient disposition. More detailed history, education, developing and facilitating a treatment plan, helping the patient to develop a relapse prevention strategy, identifying and treating other GMCs and comorbid mental disorders.

Choice of disposition is shown below:

Most restrictive ←				→ Least restrictive
Inpatient hospitalization	Residential	Partial hospitalization	Intensive outpatient	Outpatient/ self-help

Treatment settings vary widely according to the community in which a clinician practices psychiatry (Table 10-6). Such settings vary in terms of availability and treatment philosophies. Goals of treatment are generally abstinence and drug-free life including improvement in social and occupational functioning. Typically cognitive behavioral focus and choice of a treatment setting should be based on a number of factors; first and foremost the patient should be treated in the least restrictive setting that is likely to be safe and effective.

TABLE 10-6 **APPROPRIATE CHOICE OF TREATMENT SETTINGS**

Outpatient	Motivated patients with stable clinical condition and environmental supports in place who can safely participate in an outpatient program.
Partial hospital	Patients who require a more intensive setting; particularly helpful for patients leaving hospitals or residential settings who continue to display signs and symptoms of potential relapse (i.e., poor motivation, severe psychiatric comorbidity, history of relapse during immediate posthospital or postresidential period), those in high-risk environments with poor psychosocial supports. Also helpful for those who have failed in less restrictive but intensive outpatient care.
Residential	Indicated for patients who do not rise to the threshold of hospitalization but whose lives revolve around substance abuse; they lack sufficient social and vocational skills and psychosocial supports to maintain abstinence in an outpatient setting. Residential treatment of 3 months or more is associated with better long-term outcome.
Hospital	Most restrictive is an inpatient hospitalization setting. This may need to be considered for the following reasons: 1. The patient has a history of poor outpatient response and follow-through, has had multiple treatment failures on an outpatient basis. 2. The patient has a known history of dt's or other life-threatening withdrawal complications that require inpatient intervention. 3. The patient has a history of comorbid GMC that could be life-threatening if he continues to drink on an outpatient basis. 4. The patient has a history of comorbid mental illness and is also experiencing active symptoms of said illness, which increases risk on an outpatient basis (e.g., active psychosis) which would typically lead to a hospitalization even without concurrent substance use. 5. The patient is at imminent risk of self-harm or harm to others if released to a less restrictive setting.

ALCOHOL-RELATED DISORDERS

Alcoholism is an antiquated term and the savvy clinician will avoid its use in favor of DSM-IV-TR terminology. In most cultures, alcohol is the most frequently used brain depressant and a cause of considerable morbidity and mortality.

At some time in their lives, as many as 90% of adults in the United States have had some experience with alcohol; 60% of males and 30% of females have had one or more alcohol-related adverse life event (e.g., driving after consuming too much alcohol, missing school or work due to a hangover).

Alcohol use disorder includes alcohol dependence and alcohol abuse (Tables 10-7 through 10-9).

The healthy liver metabolizes alcohol at the rate of approximately 15–30 mg/hr. In the chronic alcohol-dependent individual, the rate may be closer to 30 mg/hr (which helps explain the development of tolerance since alcohol is metabolized faster) unless the alcohol-dependent patient is one of the 10% who have developed cirrhosis of the liver, in which case metabolism slows in the impaired liver (Tables 10-10 through 10-12).

TABLE 10-7 **ALCOHOL-INDUCED DISORDERS**

	DSM-IV-TR Diagnostic Criteria

Alcohol intoxication	1. Recent ingestion of alcohol.
	2. Clinically significant maladaptive behavioral or psychological changes occurring shortly after or during ingestion. These may include:
	  • Inappropriate sexual or aggressive behavior
	  • Mood lability
	  • Impaired judgment
	  • Impaired social and occupational functioning
	3. One or more of the following signs may be observed:
	  • Slow, slurred speech
	  • Incoordination
	  • Unsteady gait
	  • Nystagmus
	  • Impairment in attention or memory
	  • Stupor or coma
	4. The symptoms are not due to a GMC and are not better accounted for by another mental disorder.

Alcohol withdrawal	1. Cessation of or reduction in heavy and prolonged use of alcohol.
	2. Two or more of the following symptoms occur within several hours to a few days after Criterion 1:
	  • Autonomic hyperactivity (e.g., sweating or pulse rate greater than 100)
	  • Increased hand tremor
	  • Insomnia
	  • Nausea and vomiting
	  • Transient visual, tactile, or auditory hallucinations or illusions
	  • Psychomotor agitation
	  • Anxiety
	  • Grand mal seizures
	3. The symptoms in Criterion 2 cause clinically significant distress or impairment in social, occupational, or other important areas of functioning.
	4. The symptoms are not due to a GMC or better accounted for by another mental disorder.
	
	Specify if with perceptual disturbances.

SOURCE: Adapted from DSM-IV-TR, pp. 214–16.

TABLE 10-8 OTHER ALCOHOL-INDUCED DISORDERS

Alcohol withdrawal or intoxication delirium	DTs generally occur in those with alcohol dependence of many years' duration. Delirium tremens may result from the reduction of or cessation of alcohol intake. Can be sudden but usually within 12–36 hours with signs of autonomic instability, hallucinations, tremor, nausea and vomiting, and disorientation. Seizures, coma, death (1%) may result. Typically associated with infections, subdural hematomas, trauma, liver disease, and metabolic disorders with cause of death typically infectious fat emboli or cardiac arrhythmias usually associated with hyperkalemia, hyperpyrexia, and poor hydration.
Alcohol withdrawal seizures	On average occur 24 hours after the last drink. Typically grand mal. Hypomagnesemia.
Alcohol hallucinosis	Hallucinations, typically auditory, that persist after the alcohol-dependent individual has ceased alcohol intake; usually within 48 hours after the last drink. May last weeks to months. Continuum of clicks or humming sounds to threatening or pejorative voices.
Wernicke's encephalopathy	Mnemonic WerNICke: Nystagmus and ophthalmoplegia Incoordination, ataxia Confusion Aggressive treatment with thiamine may help to prevent progression into persisting amnestic disorder (Korsakoff's).
Alcohol-induced persisting amnesic disorder (Korsakoff's syndrome)	Thiamine (vitamin B_1) deficiency caused by malnutrition secondary to alcohol dependence. Confabulation due to memory impairment.
Alcohol-persisting dementia	Cognitive impairment affects more than memory function (distinguishes from amnestic disorder).
Alcohol use disorder NOS	Alcohol idiosyncratic intoxication.

SOURCE: Adapted from DSM-IV-TR, pp. 217–23.

TABLE 10-9 BLOOD ALCOHOL CONCENTRATIONS (BAC) CORRELATED WITH TYPICAL PRESENTATION IN NONTOLERANT ALCOHOL-INTOXICATED PATIENT

BAC (mg/dL)	Clinical Presentation
30	Attention difficulties, mild euphoria
50	Coordination problems
100	Typical drunk-driving parameter, ataxia
200	Confusion, decreased consciousness
>400	Seizure, coma, could result in death

TABLE 10-10 **ALCOHOL-RELATED DISORDERS**

Prevalence, familial pattern	Lifetime risk for general population: 15% for alcohol dependence. Risk is 3–4 times higher in close relatives of people with alcohol dependence.
Associated laboratory findings	>30 units elevation of gamma-glutamyltransferase (GGT) is a sensitive laboratory indicator of heavy drinking. >20 units of carbohydrate deficient transferring (CDT) is also associated with heavy alcohol consumption. Usually both return to normal levels within days to weeks of stopping drinking, so both are helpful in monitoring abstinence. Mean corpuscular volume (MCV) is elevated to high normal values due to the direct toxic effects of alcohol on erythropoeisis. Liver function tests (LFTs), e.g., alanine aminotransferase (ALT) and alkine phosphatase, can measure liver injury as a consequence of heavy drinking. Blood alcohol concentration (BAC) is the most direct test available to measure alcohol consumption.
Associated physical examination findings and GMC	One of the most common associated GMCs is low-grade hypertension. Cardiomyopathy and increases in lipids and cholesterol all contribute to increased risk of heart disease. GI effects include gastritis, stomach or duodenal ulcers, and, in approximately 15%, liver cirrhosis and pancreatitis. There is also an increased risk of esophageal and stomach cancer. Peripheral neuropathy may be evidenced by muscular weakness, paresthesias, and decreased peripheral sensation. Other CNS effects include cognitive deficits, severe memory impairment, and degenerative changes in the cerebellum. Alcohol-induced persisting amnesic disorder (Wernicke-Korsakoff syndrome) is the inability to encode new memory.

SOURCE: Adapted from DSM-IV-TR, pp. 217–22.

TABLE 10-11 SPECIFIC CULTURE, AGE, AND GENDER FEATURES OF ALCOHOL-RELATED DISORDERS

Culture	In the United States whites and African-Americans have similar rates of alcohol abuse and dependence. Latino males have somewhat higher rates; Latino females have lower prevalence than other females from other ethnic groups. In most Asian cultures, the overall prevalence of alcohol-related disorders is relatively low and the male-to-female ratio high. May be due to the deficiency, in as many as 50% of Japanese, Chinese, and Korean individuals, of the form of aldehyde dehydrogenase that eliminates low levels of the first breakdown product of alcohol, acetaldehyde.
Age	Elderly may need higher doses and prolonged treatment (see Table 10-12).
Gender	Pregnant women put their fetus at risk for FAS—low birthweight, poor coordination, hypotonia, neonatal irritability, retarded growth and development, craniofacial abnormalities including microcephaly, cardiovascular defects, mild to moderate retardation, childhood hyperactivity, and impaired school performance.

SOURCE: Adapted from DSM-IV-TR, pp. 219–20.

TABLE 10-12 EMERGENCY ASSESSMENT AND MANAGEMENT OF ALCOHOL DISORDERS

Biological	The acutely intoxicated patient should be monitored in a safe environment and vital signs should be monitored.

Mild to moderate withdrawal typically starts within a few hours of cessation or reduction in heavy, prolonged alcohol use; severe withdrawal typically starts within first several days of cessation or reduction of heavy, prolonged alcohol use, with symptoms that may include clouding of consciousness, difficulty in sustaining attention, disorientation, grand mal seizure, reparatory alkalosis, and fever. Fewer than 5% of individuals with alcohol withdrawal develop severe symptoms and fewer than 3% develop grand mal seizures.

Generalized support, reassurance, and frequent monitoring are sufficient for approximately two-thirds of the patients with mild to moderate withdrawal symptoms. Patients in more severe withdrawal and those who develop hallucinations require pharmacological intervention. Supportive measures include hydration and nutrition.

Baseline labs if indicated, Mg level, BAC serially, thiamine. For most patients the equivalent of 600 mg/day of chlordiazepoxide is the maximum dose. The total dose necessary to suppress autonomic hyperactivity in the first 24 hours, i.e., the stabilization dose, is then given in four divided doses the following day, after which the dose can usually be tapered over 3–5 days, with monitoring for reemergence of symptoms. Short-acting benzodiazepines (e.g., lorazepam) are preferable for patients with severe hepatic disease, the elderly, and patients with cognitive disorders, since these agents have the advantage of being metabolized and excreted primarily via the kidneys. Plus there are no intermediary metabolites to accumulate and there is IM and IV availability. However, their short half-lives may mean an increased frequency of dispensation. If signs of withdrawal are noted, beta-blockers (e.g., propanolol, 10 mg PO q6h, or atenolol C) can help reduce autonomic nervous system hyperactivity and, when used with benzodiazepines, may allow use of lower doses of BZs and thus reduce the sedation and cognitive impairment often associated with BZ use.

Clonidine, an alpha-adrenergic agonist (0.5 b.i.d. or t.i.d.), may also reduce autonomic signs of hyperactivity. Neither should be used alone, however, to manage alcohol withdrawal symptoms due to their lack of efficacy in preventing seizures.

Barbiturates may also be useful in reducing withdrawal symptoms in patients refractory to BZs.

In patients manifesting delirium, delusions, or hallucinations, haloperidol, 0.5–0.2 mg IM q2h, may be needed. Usually less than 10 mg is given in 24 hours as an adjunct to BZs since antipsychotic agents are not effective for treating the underlying withdrawal state.

(continued)

Anticonvulsant use is controversial. If patients have a prior history of withdrawal-related seizures, BZs are generally effective. But if they have a history of non-withdrawal-related seizure disorder, start their anticonvulsant or continue. IM magnesium sulfate has also been used for preventing withdrawal seizures.

Comorbid psychiatric and general medical disorders: If there are comorbid depression or anxiety disorders, consider antidepressant agents with low potential for lethality in overdose situations and dispensing limited amounts of medications. Most observe over 3–4 weeks during an alcohol-free period before diagnosing a comorbid psychiatric disorder unless there is a compelling reason to initiate earlier treatment (e.g., in depressed patients with a prior history of major depression unrelated to periods of alcohol use and/or strong family history of affective disorder). (More likely to have a comorbid primary depression that should be treated as soon as detoxification is completed.)

Use of BZs for alcohol-dependent patients is controversial, since there is a high potential for abuse. Beta-blockers and buspirone may be preferable since they have no cross-tolerance with ethanol or other CNS depressants and minimal abuse potential. Clonazepam or other long-acting benzodiazepines may be utilized.

Treatment of comorbid GMCs is focused on restoring physiological homeostasis, with thiamine (50–100 mg/day IM or IV), fluids, benzodiazepines, and other medications. In the elderly: one study found that patients aged 58–77 required higher BZ doses during a 5-day detoxification and may need a longer determination period than younger patients.

Residential or hospital setting would be appropriate for patients:
- In severe withdrawal
- With a prior history of DTs
- With a documented history of heavy, prolonged alcohol use and high tolerances (places them at risk for a complicated withdrawal syndrome)
- Concurrently abusing other drugs
- With comorbid GMC or psychiatric disorder
- Who repeatedly fail to cooperate with or benefit from outpatient detoxification

Psychosocial	Supportive
	CBT
	Behavioral
	Marital/family/group therapy
	Self-help groups such as AA
	Once stabilized, CD referral

AMPHETAMINE-RELATED DISORDERS

The class of amphetamine and amphetamine-like substances includes all substances with a substituted-phenyethylamine structure such as amphetamine, dextroamphetamine, and methamphetamine ("speed") as well as methylphenidate or agents used as appetite suppressants. How are these similar to cocaine? Both are stimulants. They are different from cocaine in that cocaine is mostly obtained illegally and has a local anesthetic activity that increases cocaine's risk for inducing certain GMCs such as cardiac arrhythmias and seizures. The psychoactive effects of amphetamine-like substances last longer than those of cocaine and the peripheral sympathomimetic effects may be more potent (Tables 10-13 through 10-15).

TABLE 10-13   AMPHETAMINE OR AMPHETAMINE-LIKE RELATED DISORDERS

Prevalence, familial pattern	Patterns of use differ between locales (e.g., high rate in southern California. Surveys measure how many have used the drug.). In 1997 high-school seniors reported that 16% had ever used amphetamine-like drugs but it is not known how many met criteria for abuse or dependence.
Associated descriptive features and mental disorders	Acute amphetamine intoxication is sometimes associated with rambling speech, headache, transient ideas of reference, and tinnitus. More severe intoxication can produce paranoid ideation, auditory hallucinations in a clear sensorium, and tactile hallucinations (e.g., formication, or a feeling of bugs under the skin). Insight is typically intact. Extreme anger, mood lability, irritability, anhedonia, weight loss, and impaired personal hygiene may be seen with sustained amphetamine dependence.
Associated laboratory findings	Urine tests usually remain positive for only 1–3 days even after a binge.
Associated physical examination findings and GMC	Adverse pulmonary effects are seen less often that with cocaine because substances in this class are smoked fewer times per day. Seizures, HIV infection, malnutrition, gunshot or knife wounds, nosebleeds, and CV problems may be seen as presenting complaints in those with amphetamine-related disorders.

SOURCE: Adapted from DSM-IV-TR, pp. 223–31.

TABLE 10-14   SPECIFIC CULTURE, AGE, AND GENDER FEATURES OF AMPHETAMINE-RELATED DISORDERS

Culture	IV use more common among lower socioeconomic status.
Age	More common among young adults.
Gender	Male to female ratio is 3 or 4:1 with IV use; 1:1 with non-IV use.

SOURCE: Adapted from DSM-IV-TR, p. 229.

TABLE 10-15 EMERGENCY ASSESSMENT AND MANAGEMENT OF AMPHETAMINE DISORDERS

Biological	Hx + PE, collateral info, medical records.
	R/O GMCs:
	Cocaine intoxication can produce hypertension, tachycardia, seizures, and/or paranoid delusions.
	Acute agitation may require sedation with benzodiazepines, or antipsychotic may be necessary.
Psychosocial	Supportive.
	CBT and behavioral therapies are recommended with moderate clinical confidence.
	Self-help groups.

CAFFEINE-RELATED DISORDERS

The authors include this as a likely problematic, clinically relevant situation that is often overlooked in search of other disorders to explain symptoms. The authors think it is important to remember that a high proportion of the mentally ill overconsume caffeine relative to the general population (Tables 10-16, 10-17).

EMERGENCY ASSESSMENT AND MANAGEMENT OF CAFFEINE DISORDERS

See general management guidelines.

TABLE 10-16 CAFFEINE-RELATED DISORDERS

Prevalence, familial pattern	80–85% of adults consume caffeine in any given year. Among consumers of caffeine, 85% or more use a caffeine-containing beverage at least once a week, an average of 200 mg/day. Typically caffeine intake is elevated among those who smoke, drink, and use other substances.
Associated descriptive features and mental disorders	Mild sensory disturbance (e.g., ringing in the ears and flashes of light at higher doses). Large doses can increase heart rate, while smaller doses decrease it. Excessive caffeine use is associated with mood, eating, psychotic, sleep and substance-related disorders. Anxiety-disordered persons are likely to avoid.
Associated laboratory findings	No specific laboratory findings.
Associated physical examination findings and GMC	Agitation, restlessness, sweating, tachycardia, flushed face, and increased bowel motility. Heavy prolonged used is associated with the development of exacerbation of anxiety and somatic symptoms such as cardiac arrhythmias, and GI pain or diarrhea. Acute doses exceeding 10 g of caffeine (brewed coffee has 100–140 mg/80 ounces) may induce grand mal seizures and respiratory failure resulting in death.

SOURCE: Adapted from DSM-IV-TR, pp. 231–34.

TABLE 10-17 SPECIFIC CULTURE, AGE, AND GENDER FEATURES OF CAFFEINE-RELATED DISORDERS

Culture	Average caffeine intake in most of the developing world is less than 50 mg/day vs. 400 mg/day in Sweden, the United Kingdom, and other European nations.
Age	Caffeine consumption increases during the 20s and often decreases after age 65.
Gender	Intake greater in males than females.

SOURCE: Adapted from DSM-IV-TR, p. 233.

CANNABIS-RELATED DISORDERS

The cannabinoid primarily responsible for the psychoactive effects of cannabis is delta-9-tetrahydrocannabinol (also known as THC or delta-9-THC). It acts on CB1 and CB2 cannabinoid receptors that are found throughout the CNS. Synthetic delta-9-THC is used for general medication conditions (e.g., nausea and vomiting caused by chemotherapy, anorexia and weight loss in individuals with AIDS) (Table 10-18).

EMERGENCY ASSESSMENT AND MANAGEMENT OF CANNABIS DISORDERS

See general management guidelines.

TABLE 10-18 **CANNABIS-RELATED DISORDERS**

Prevalence, familial pattern	Most widely used illicit psychoactive substance in the United States. Age span with the highest lifetime prevalence was 26–34 years (50%). Surveys have assessed patterns of use rather than measured how may individuals met criteria for dependence or abuse.
Associated descriptive features and mental disorders	Often used with other substances. Regular use associated with mild forms of depression, anxiety, or irritability in one-third of users. At high doses, psychoactive effects may cause severe panic attacks and/or paranoia. Depersonalization and derealization may occur.
Associated laboratory findings	Urine tests—because these substances are fat-soluble, persist in bodily fluids for extended periods of time, and are expected slowly, routine urine tests for individuals who use cannabis can be positive for 7–10 days; urine of individuals with heavy use of cannabis may test positive for 2–4 weeks. Other biological alterations can be temporary, dose-related suppression of immunological function, suppressed secretion of testosterone and luteininzing hormone. Acute cannibinoid intoxication can cause diffuse slowing of background activity on EEG and REM suppression.
Associated physical examination findings and GMC	Since cannabis smoke is highly irritating to the nasopharynx and bronchial lining, increased risk for chronic cough, sinusitis, pharyngitis, emphysema, and pulmonary dysplasia may occur with chronic heavy use. Sometimes associated with weight gain.

SOURCE: Adapted from DSM-IV-TR, pp. 234–41.

COCAINE-RELATED DISORDERS

Cocaine is the active ingredient of the coca plant of Central and South America. Cocaine is consumed in several preparations (e.g., coca leaves, coca paste, cocaine hydrochloride, and cocaine alkaloids such as freebase and crack). Cocaine hydrochloride powder is usually snorted or dissolved in water and injected IV. Freebasing involved separating or "freeing" the cocaine from its hydrochloride base by heating it with ether, ammonia, or some other volatile substance and then smoking it.

Crack is a cocaine alkaloid that is extracted from its powdered hydrochloride salt by mixing it with sodium bicarbonate and allowing it to dry into rocks. These rocks are easily vaporized and inhaled, thus producing an almost instantaneous and highly addictive high.

Cocaine use disorders include cocaine dependence and cocaine abuse. See "Review of DSM-IV-TR Criteria" (Tables 10-19 through 10-22).

TABLE 10-19 COCAINE-INDUCED DISORDERS

	Essential Features
Cocaine intoxication	Clinically significant maladaptive behavioral or psychological changes that develop during or shortly after use of cocaine. These include: • Euphoria or affective blunting • Increased sociability • Hypervigilance • Interpersonal sensitivity • Anxiety, tension, or anger • Steretyped behaviors • Impaired judgment • Impaired social or occupational functioning Two or more of the following develop during or shortly after cocaine use: • Tachycardia or bradycardia • Papillary dilation • Elevated or lowered blood pressure • Perspiration or chills • Nausea or vomiting • Evidence of weight loss • Psychomotor agitation or retardation • Muscular weakness, respiratory depression, chest pain, or cardiac arrythmias • Confusion, seizures, dyskinesias, dystonias, or coma
	DSM-IV-TR Diagnostic Criteria

Cocaine withdrawal	1. Cessation of or reduction of cocaine use that has been heavy and prolonged.
	2. Dsyphoric mood and two or more of the following physiological changes developing within a few hours to several days:
	  • Fatigue
	  • Vivid unpleasant dreams
	  • Increased appetite
	  • Hypersomnia or insomnia
	  • Psychomotor retardation or agitation
	3. These symptoms cause clinically significant distress or impairment in social, occupational, or other important areas of functioning.
	4. The symptoms are not due to a GMC and are not better accounted for by another mental disorder.

Other cocaine-induced disorders	Cocaine intoxication delirium Cocaine-induced psychotic disorder Cocaine-induced mood disorder Cocaine-induced anxiety disorder Cocaine-induced sexual dysfunction Cocaine-induced sleep disorder

SOURCE: Adapted from DSM-IV-TR, pp. 241–50.

TABLE 10-20 **COCAINE-RELATED DISORDERS**

Prevalence	Lifetime prevalence estimated at 2%.
Associated descriptive features and mental disorders	Cocaine is a short-acting drug that produces rapid effects on the CNS especially when taken IV, snorted, or smoked in crack form. It produces an instant feeling of well-being, confidence, and euphoria. Acute intoxication may also be associated with rambling speech, headache, transient ideas of reference, and tinnitus. Individuals who develop cocaine dependence may become driven to obtain the drug, resorting to spending thousands of dollars, engaging in prostitution, and other criminal activities in order to get the drug. Comorbid disorders may include MDD, anxiety disorders, eating disorders, cocaine-induced psychotic disorder that resembles schizophrenia, paranoid type. Other substance dependence or abuse, especially with alcohol, cannabis, heroin, and sedatives. Hypnotics, anxiolytics. Moreover, PTSD, ASPD, ADHD, and pathological gambling may also be associated with cocaine dependence.
Associated laboratory findings	Benzoylecgonine, a metabolite of cocaine that remains in the urine for 1–3 days after a single dose, 7–12 days after repeated high doses. Mildly elevated liver function tests, hepatitis, STDs, TB, pnemonitis, or pneuthorax may co-occur.
Associated physical examination findings and GMC	GMCs may predictably occur specific to the route of administration of the drug (e.g., snorting may lead to erosion of nasopharyngeal tissue and frequent nosebleeds, sinusitis acute and chronic, and perforated nasal septum; smoking may lead to chronic bronchitis and cough, pneumonia, pneumothorax; injection may lead to vasculitis, infection at the injection site, sepsis, HIV from sharing contaminated needles, and promiscuous sexual behavior that may accompany). Other STDs, hepatitis, and TB and other lung infections. Since cocaine has an appetite-suppressant effect, malnutrition and weight loss may occur. Chest pain, pneumothorax from performing valsalva maneuvers to better absorb inhaled cocaine. Cocaine's ability to increase BP, cause vasoconstriction, and/or alter the electrical activity of the heart may lead to MI, palpitations and arrhythmias, sudden death from respiratory or cardiac arrest, and stroke. Seizures. Traumatic injuries due to violent behavior. Pregnancy: female user may suffer with irregularities in placental blood flow, abruption placenta, premature labor and delivery, and increased prevalence of infants with very low birthweights.

SOURCE: Adapted from DSM-IV-TR, pp. 241–50.

TABLE 10-21 SPECIFIC CULTURE, AGE, AND GENDER FEATURES OF COCAINE-RELATED DISORDERS

Culture	Cocaine use started in the 1970s among the affluent, but shifted to lower socioeconomic groups living in large urban areas. Roughly similar rates have been noted across different racial groups.
Age	Individuals between ages 26 and 34. Highest rates of lifetime use: 21% cocaine; 4% crack.
Gender	Males are more commonly affected than females, with a male-to-female ratio of 1.5–2.0:1.

SOURCE: Adapted from DSM-IV-TR, p. 248.

TABLE 10-22 EMERGENCY ASSESSMENT AND MANAGEMENT OF COCAINE USE DISORDERS

Biological	Hx + PE, collateral info, medical records. R/O GMCs: Cocaine intoxication can produce hypertension, tachycardia, seizures, and/or paranoid delusions. Acute agitation may require sedation with benzodiazepines, or antipsychotic may be necessary.
Psychosocial	Supportive/encouraging. CBT and behavioral therapies have received moderate clinical confidence. Self-help groups.

HALLUCINOGEN-RELATED DISORDERS

This group of substances includes: ergot and related compounds like lysergic diethyamide (LSD), morning glory seeds, phenylalkylamines [mescaline, "STP" (2.5-dimethoxy-4-methylamphetamine), and MDMA (3,4-methylenedioxymethamphetamine, also called Ecstasy), indole alkaloids (psilocybin, DMT), methyltyrptamine], and miscellaneous other compounds. The disorders are divided into hallucinogen use disorders, disorders of hallucinogen dependence and hallucinogen abuse (see general criteria), and hallucinogen-induced disorders (Tables 10-23 through 10-25).

MANAGEMENT OF HALLUCINOGEN DISORDERS

See general management guidelines.

TABLE 10-23   HALLUCINOGEN-INDUCED DISORDERS

	DSM-IV-TR Diagnostic Criteria
Hallucinogen intoxication	Clinically significant maladaptive behavioral or psychological changes that developed during or shortly after hallucinogen use. These may include: • Marked anxiety or depression • Ideas of reference • Fear of losing one's mind • Paranoid ideation • Impaired judgment • Impaired social or occupational functioning Perceptual changes occurring during a state of full wakefulness and alertness that developed during or shortly after hallucinogen use. These may include: • Subjective intensification of perceptions • Depersonalization • Derealization • Illusions • Hallucinations • Syntesthesias Two or more of the following signs may develop: • Papillary dilation • Tachycardia • Sweating • Palpitation • Blurring of vision • Tremors • Incoordination The symptoms are not due to a GMC and are not better accounted for by another mental disorder.
Hallucinogen persisting perception disorder (flashbacks)*	The reexperiencing, following cessation of use of a hallucinogen, of one or more of the perceptual symptoms that were experienced while intoxicated with the hallucinogen. These may include: • Geometric hallucinations • False perceptions of movement in the peripheral visual fields • Flashes of color • Intensified colors • Trails of images of moving objects • Positive afterimages • Halos around objects • Marcopsia • Micropsia The symptoms are not due to a GMC and are not better accounted for by another mental disorder.

*There is not a documented clinically significant withdrawal syndrome that occurs with hallucinogens. However, a hallucinogen persisting perception disorder can occur.

Source: Adapted from DSM-IV-TR, pp. 250–57.

TABLE 10-24 HALLUCINOGEN-RELATED DISORDERS

Prevalence, familial pattern	Lifetime prevalence rates of hallucinogen abuse or dependence in the United States are estimated to be about 0.6%.
Associated descriptive features and mental disorders	Perceptual distortions and impaired judgment may result in injuries or fatalities. Environmental factors and the personality and expectations of the individual using the hallucinogen may contribute to the nature and severity of the hallucinogen intoxication, or "trip." May co-occur with preexisting adolescent conduct disorder or adult ASPD.
Associated laboratory findings	Can be confirmed with urine toxicology.

SOURCE: Adapted from DSM-IV-TR, pp. 250–57.

TABLE 10-25 SPECIFIC CULTURE, AGE, AND GENDER FEATURES OF HALLUCINOGEN-RELATED DISORDERS

Culture	Hallucinogens may be used as part of established religious practices, such as peyote in the Native American Church. Within the United States, there are regional differences and changes in patterns of use over the decades. Hallucinogens came into vogue in the United States in the 1960s. In the 1990s there has been a resurgence of use of LSD and MDMA, a mixed hallucinogen-amphetamine drug.
Age	Hallucinogen intoxication usually first occurs in adolescence, and younger users may tend to experience more disruptive emotions.
Gender	Hallucinogen use and intoxication appear to be three times more common among males than among females.

SOURCE: Adapted from DSM-IV-TR, p. 255.

INHALANT-RELATED DISORDERS

These include those disorders induced by inhaling the aliphatic and aromatic hydrocarbons found in substances such as gasoline, glue, paint thinners, and spray paints. Halogenated hydrocarbons found in cleaners, typewriter correction fluid, spray-can propellants, and other volatile compounds conatin esters, ketones, and glycols. Active ingredients may include toluene, benzene, acetone, and tetrachloroethylene. Most compounds that are inhaled are a mixture of several substances that can produce psychoactive effects. These volatile substances are available in a wide variety of commercial products. All are capable of producing dependence, abuse, and intoxica-tion. Several methods are used to inhale intoxicating vapors. Most commonly, a rag soaked with the substance is applied to the mouth and nose, and vapors are breathed in; this is called "huffing." Also, the substance may be placed in a paper or plastic bag and inhaled; this is called "bagging." Substances may also be inhaled directly from containers or from aerosol sprayed in the mouth or nose. Heating compounds to accelerate vaporization and absorption also occurs. No clinically meaningful withdrawal syndrome is established in humans (Tables 10-26 through 10-28).

MANAGEMENT OF INHALANT USE DISORDERS

See general management guidelines.

TABLE 10-26 INHALANT-INDUCED DISORDERS

	DSM-IV-TR Diagnostic Criteria
Inhalant intoxication	1. Recent intentional use or short-term, high-dose exposure to volatile inhalants (excluding anesthetic gases and short-acting vasodilators).
	2. Clinically significant maladaptive behavioral or psychological changes that developed during, or shortly after, use of or exposure to volatile inhalants. These may include:
	• Belligerence
	• Assaultiveness
	• Apathy
	• Impaired judgment
	• Impaired social or occupational functioning
	3. Two or more of the following signs, developing during, or shortly after, inhalant use or exposure:
	• Dizziness
	• Nystagmus
	• Incoordiantion
	• Slurred speech
	• Unsteady gait
	• Lethargy
	• Depressed reflexes
	• Psychomotor retardation
	• Tremor
	• Generalized muscle weakness
	• Blurred vision or diplopia
	• Stupor or coma
	• Euphoria
	4. The symptoms are not due to a GMC and are not better accounted for by another mental disorder.

SOURCE: Adapted from DSM-IV-TR, pp. 257–64.

TABLE 10-27   **INHALANT-RELATED DISORDERS**

Prevalence, familial pattern	Unknown. Surveys measuring patterns of use rather than disorders found that: 6% of people in the United States acknowledged ever having used inhalants with the highest prevalence in the 18–25-year-olds.
Associated descriptive features and mental disorders	Additional psychiatric symptoms may include: • Hallucinations—auditory, visual, or tactile • Other perceptual disorders such as macropsia, micropsia, illusional misperceptions, alterations in time perception • Delusions • Anxiety • Also school, social, and work problems
Associated laboratory findings	Direct assay for inhalants is not available. However, a metabolite of toluene, hippuric acid, is excreted in the urine and a ratio greater than 1 in relation to creatinine might be suggestive of toluene use. Damage to muscles, kidneys, liver, and other organs may be evidenced in general chemistry.
Associated physical examination findings and GMC	Odor of paint or solvents. Residue of same on clothing or skin. Glue sniffer's rash around the mouth or nose and conjuctival irritation. Trauma due to disinhibited behavior. Burns due to flammable nature. Nonspecific respiratory findings, include: • Upper or lower-airway irritation • Increased airway resistance, pulmonary hypertension acute respiratory distress, coughing, sinus discharge, dyspnea, rales, or rhonchi • Headache • Generalized weakness • Abdominal pain • Nausea • Vomiting • Central and peripheral nervous system damage • Cerebral atrophy, cerebellar degeneration • White matter lesions resulting in cranial nerve or pyramidal tract signs • Hepatitis, cirrhosis, metallic acidosis Chronic renal failure, hepatorenal syndrome, bone marrow suppression especially with benzene and trichoroethlene. Some inhalants (e.g., methylene chloride) may be metabolized to carbon monoxide and death may occur from respiratory or cardiovascular depression. Sudden-sniffing death may result from acute arrhythmia, hypoxia, or electrolyte abnormalities.

SOURCE: Adapted from DSM-IV-TR, pp. 257–64.

TABLE 10-28 **SPECIFIC CULTURE, AGE, AND GENDER FEATURES OF INHALANT-RELATED DISORDERS**

Culture	Rural Alaskan-native children, almost 50% in isolated villages, have at some time used solvents to get high.
Age	Low cost and easy availability make these drugs often the first drugs of experimentation for youth. May begin at ages 9–12, peaks in adolescence, and is less common after age 35. Most commonly used by adolescents in a group setting.
Gender	Males account for 70–80% of inhalant-related emergency-room visits. Rates were higher among impoverished children and young adults.

SOURCE: Adapted from DSM-IV-TR, p. 262.

OPIOID-RELATED DISORDERS

The opioids include:

- Natural opioids (morphine)
- Semisynthetics (heroin)
- Synthetics (with morphine-like action, (including codeine, hydromorphone, methadone, oxycodone, mepiridine, fetanyl)
- Mixed opionate agonists and antagonists include pentazocine, buprenorphine

Opioids are prescribed as:

- Analgesics
- Anesthetics
- Antidiarrheal agents
- Cough suppressants

Heroin is injected, smoked, or snorted. Fentanyl is injected. Cough suppressants and antidiarrheal agents are taken orally.

Opioid use disorders include opioid dependence and opioid abuse (Tables 10-29 through 10-32).

TABLE 10-29   **OPIOID-INDUCED DISORDERS**

	DSM-IV-TR Criteria
Opioid intoxication	1. Recent use of an opioid. 2. Clinically maladaptive behavioral or psychological changes that developed during, or shortly after, opioid use. These include: • Initial euphoria followed by apathy • Dypshoria • Psychomotor agitiation or retardation • Impaired judgment • Impaired social or occupational functioning 3. Pupillary constriction or pupillary dilation due to anoxia (from severe overdose) and one or more of the following signs developing during, or shortly after, opioid use: • Drowsiness or coma • Slurred speech • Impairment in attention or memory 4. The symptoms are not due to a GMC and are not better accounted for by another mental disorder.
Opioid withdrawal	1. Either of the following: • Cessation of or reduction in opioid use that has been heavy and prolonged several weeks or longer. • Administration of an opioid antagonist after a period of opioid use. 2. Three or more of the following developing within minutes to several days after Criterion 1: • Dysphoric mood • Nausea and vomiting • Muscle aches • Lacrimation or rhinorrhea • Papillary dilation, piloerection, or sweating • Diarrhea • Yawning • Fever • Insomnia 3. The symptoms in Criterion 2 cause clinically significant distress or impairment in social, occupational, or other important areas of functioning. 4. The symptoms are not due to a general medical condition and are not better accounted for by another mental disorder.

SOURCE: Adapted from DSM-IV-TR, pp. 271–73.

TABLE 10-30 **OPIOID-RELATED DISORDERS**

Prevalence, familial pattern	1996 national survey of drug use reported that 6.7% of men and 4.5% of women use opioids.
Associated descriptive features and mental disorders	Drug-related crimes Divorce, unemployment, or irregular employment Depression and insomnia may occur. ASPD PTSD History of conduct disorder in childhood or adolescence has been identified as a significant risk factor for substance-related disorders, especially opioid dependence.
Associated laboratory findings	Urine tests remain positive for most opioids for 12–36 hours after administration. Longer-acting opioids (e.g., methadone and LAAM) can be identified in urine for several days. Fentanyl is not detected by standard urine tests. Screening tests for hepatitis A, B, and C is positive in as many as 80–90% of intravenous users for either hepatitis antigen (signifying active infection) or hepatitis antibody (signifying past infection.)
Associated physical examination findings and GMC	Acute and chronic opioid use is associated with a lack of secretions causing dry mouth and nose, slowing of gastrointestinal activity, and constipation. Visual acuity may be impaired due to papillary constriction. IV use causes tracks (sclerosis of veins at injection sites). Veins in legs, neck, and groin may be used. Skin popping by injection directly into subcutaneous tissue can lead to cellulitis, abscesses, and circular-appearing scars from healed skin lesions. Infections, tuberculosis, HIV infection. As high as 60% among persons dependent on heroin in some areas of the United States. In addition to infections like cellulitis, hepatitis, HIV, tuberculosis, and endocarditis, opioid dependence is associated with a death rate as high as 1.5–2% per year. Death results from overdose, accidents, injuries, AIDS, and other general medical complications. Violence associated with buying or selling drugs. Physiological dependence on opioids may occur in about half of the infants born to females with opioid dependence, which can produce severe withdrawal syndrome.

SOURCE: Adapted from DSM-IV-TR, pp. 270–77.

TABLE 10-31   **SPECIFIC CULTURE, AGE, AND GENDER FEATURES OF**
OPIOID-RELATED DISORDERS

Culture	In the late 1800s and early 1900s, opioid dependence was seen more often among white middle-class, especially women. Since the 1920s, increased use in minority groups living in economically impoverished areas.
Age	Increasing age associated with decreasing prevalence. "Maturing out."
Gender	Males are more commonly affected with the male-to-female ratio typically being 1.5:1 for opioids other than heroin (i.e., available by prescription), and 3:1 for heroin.

SOURCE: Adapted from DSM-IV-TR, p. 276.

TABLE 10-32 EMERGENCY ASSESSMENT AND MANAGEMENT OF OPIOID-INDUCED DISORDERS

Biological

Severe opioid overdose marked by respiratory depression and is life-threatening. Naloxone can reverse.

There are pharmacological strategies in general use to manage withdrawal:

1. Methadone substitution 10–40 mg. Will stabilize most patients and control abstinence symptoms.
2. Clonidine-assisted detoxification—Clonidine is a nonopioid antihypertensive agent that acts by stimulating midbrain alpha-2-adrenergic receptors, thereby reducing the noradrenergic hyperactivity that accounts for many of the symptoms of opioid withdrawal. First day of treatment is typically 0.1–0.3 mg t.i.d. usually sufficient to suppress signs of opioid withdrawal, without causing hypotension and oversedation. If the BP falls below 90/60 mmHg, the next dose should be withheld. Not FDA approved for the treatment of opioid withdrawal. However, advantages include: no postmethadone rebound in withdrawal symptoms, no opioid-like tolerance or physical dependence. Also could consider giving outpatients a 3-day supply of clonidine for unsupervised use but no more is recommended since clonidine overdoses can be life-threatening. Disadvantages include hypotension, sedation/insomnia.
3. Clonidine-naltrexone ultrarapid withdrawal—Naltrexone-precipitated withdrawal is avoided by pretreating the patient with clonidine. Monitoring for withdrawal particularly on Day 1 and careful BP monitoring throughout the process.
4. Buprenorphine—a partial opioid agonist. At 2–4 mg sublingually, the drug blocks the signs and symptoms of opioid withdrawal.

Others include sedative-hypnotics, BZs. Antihistamines, acute opioid withdrawal not typically treated except with benzodiazepines. Facilitate treatment in a specialized treatment program that may include agonist substitution therapy with methadone (dose range of 10–20 mg/day to >60 mg/day to block craving and suppress opioid withdrawal symptoms) or LAAM (long-acting as prescribed in doses of 20–140 mg; average 60 mg) 3 times per week.

Opioid antagonist treatment: naltrexone (typically 100 mg PO on Monday and Wednesday and 150 mg on Friday). Alternative to methadone or LAAM.

With gradual tapering. Clonidine to suppress withdrawal symptoms. Clonidine-naltrexone detoxification: monitor for the presence of comorbid substance use disorders.

Comorbid psychiatric disorders should also be treated with attention to avoiding medications with high abuse potential and possible drug-drug interactions between opioids and other psychoactive substances. BZs with a slower onset of action are preferred since they also have a lower abuse potential.

(continued)

	Comorbid GMCs.
	Pregnant patients: One-half of infants born to women with opioid dependence are physiologically dependent on opioids and may experience withdrawal that requires pharmacological intervention. Methadone maintenance is indicated in pregnant patients who lack the motivation and support to remain drug-free during pregnancy.
Psychosocial	Supportive/encouraging/instill hope.
	Therapeutic communities.

PHENCYCLIDINE-RELATED DISORDERS

Phencyclidines or phencyclidine-like substances include phencyclidine (PCP, Sernylan) and the less potent ketamine, cyclohexamine, and dizocipine. These were first developed in the 1950s as dissociative anesthetics. By the 1960s they were street drugs. Phencyclidine can be taken PO or IV or smoked. Since symptoms of phencyclidine have not been found clinically significant, there is no DSM-IV-TR diagnosis of phencyclidine withdrawal. Peak effects occur about 2 hours after oral doses and typically resolve after 8–20 hours, whereas signs and symptoms of severe intoxication may persist for several days. Phencyclidine psychotic disorder may persist for weeks (Tables 10-33 through 10-35).

EMERGENCY ASSESSMENT AND MANAGEMENT OF PHENCYCLIDINE DISORDERS

See general management guidelines.

TABLE 10-33 **PHENCYCLIDINE-INDUCED DISORDERS**

	DSM-IV-TR Diagnostic Criteria
Phencyclidine intoxication	1. Recent ingestion of phencyclidine.
	2. Clinically significant maladaptive behavioral changes shortly after or during the ingestion of phencyclidine. The symptoms cause clinically significant distress or impairment in social, occupational, and other important activities. These may include: • Anger • Irritability • Belligerence • Aggression • Impaired judgment • Impaired insight
	3. Within an hour (less when smoked, snorted, or used IV) two of the following symptoms may occur: • Nystagmus (vertical or horizontal) • Hypertension or tachycardia • Numbness or diminished responsiveness to pain • Ataxia • Dysarthria • Muscle rigidity • Seizures or coma • Hyperacusis
	4. The symptoms are not due to a GMC and are not better accounted for by another mental disorder. Specify if with perceptual disturbances.

SOURCE: Adapted from DSM-IV-TR, p. 280.

TABLE 10-34 PHENCYCLIDINE-RELATED DISORDERS

Prevalence, familial pattern	Prevalence in the general population is unknown. Drug surveys measuring patterns of use rather than disorders show that the highest lifetime prevalence was in those aged 26–34 (4%).
Associated descriptive features and mental disorders	Phencyclidine intoxication may lead to delirium, coma, psychotic symptoms, or catatonic mutism with posturing. Violence, agitation, and bizarre behavior such as confused wandering may occur. These may lead to hospitalizations, emergency-room visits, and arrests for bizarre conduct or for fighting. Job, family, social, legal problems may result. Conduct disorder in adolescents and ASPD in adults associated. Comorbid dependence of other substances such as alcohol, amphetamines, and cocaine.
Associated laboratory findings	Phencyclidine may be detectable in urine for several weeks after the end of prolonged or very high dose use because of its high lipid solubility. Creatine phosphokinase (CPK) and serum glutamic-oxaloacetic transaminase (SGOT) are often elevated, reflecting muscle damage.
Associated physical examination findings and GMC	Cardiovascular and neurological toxicity: PCP intoxication often present with nystagmus or elevated blood pressure. May be physical evidence of injuries from fights, falls. IV phencyclidine users may present with needle tracks, infections, HIV. Drowning has been reported. Respiratory problems, rhabdomyolysis with renal impairment is seen in about 2% of individuals who seek emergency care.

SOURCE: Adapted from DSM-IV-TR, pp. 280–84.

TABLE 10-35 SPECIFIC CULTURE, AGE, AND GENDER FEATURES OF PHENCYCLIDINE-RELATED DISORDERS

Culture	Prevalence appears to be highest among ethnic minorities.
Age	Between ages 20 and 40.
Gender	Males compose about three-quarters of those with phencyclidine-related emergency-room visits.

SOURCE: Adapted from DSM-IV-TR, p. 282.

SEDATIVE-, HYPNOTIC-, OR ANXIOLYTIC-RELATED DISORDERS

The sedative, hypnotic, and anxiolytic substances include the following:

- Benzodiazepines
- Benzodiazepine-like drugs (zolpidem and zaleplon)
- Barbiturates (secobarbital)
- Barbiturate-like drugs (methaqualone)
- Carbamates (gluthethimide, meprobamate)

This class includes all prescription sleeping medications and almost all prescription anti-anxiety medications. They are available both by prescription and from illegal sources.

Nonbenzodiazepine antianxiety drugs are not included in this class. Like alcohol, these agents are CNS depressants and can produce similar substance-induced and substance use disorders (Tables 10-36 through 10-38).

EMERGENCY ASSESSMENT AND MANAGEMENT OF SEDATIVE-, HYPNOTIC-, OR ANXIOLYTIC-RELATED DISORDERS

See previous section on alcohol-related disorders.

TABLE 10-36   **SEDATIVE-, HYPNOTIC-, OR ANXIOLYTIC-INDUCED DISORDERS**

	DSM-IV-TR Diagnostic Criteria

Sedative, hypnotic, or anxiolytic intoxication	1. Recent ingestion of a sedative, hypnotic, or anxiolytic.
	2. Clinically significant maladaptive behavioral or psychological changes occurring shortly after or during ingestion. These may include:
	  • Inappropriate sexual or aggressive behavior
	  • Mood lability
	  • Impaired judgment
	  • Impaired social and occupational functioning
	3. One or more of the following signs may be observed:
	  • Slow, slurred speech
	  • Incoordination
	  • Unsteady gait
	  • Nystagmus
	  • Impairment in attention or memory
	  • Stupor or coma
	4. The symptoms are not due to a GMC and are not better accounted for by another mental disorder.

Sedative, hypnotic, or anxiolytic withdrawal	1. Cessation of (or reduction in) heavy and prolonged use of a sedative, hypnotic, or anxiolytic agent.
	2. Two or more of the following symptoms occur within several hours to a few days after Criterion 1:
	  • Autonomic hyperactivity (e.g., sweating or pulse rate greater than 100)
	  • Increased hand tremor
	  • Insomnia
	  • Nausea and vomiting
	  • Transient visual, tactile, or auditory hallucinations or illusions
	  • Psychomotor agitation
	  • Anxiety
	  • Grand mal seizures
	3. The symptoms in Criterion 2 cause clinically significant distress or impairment in social, occupational, or other important areas of functioning.
	4. The symptoms are not due to a GMC or better accounted for by another mental disorder.
	Specify if with perceptual disturbances.

SOURCE: Adapted from DSM-IV-TR, pp. 284–93.

TABLE 10-37   SEDATIVE-, HYPNOTIC-, OR ANXIOLYTIC-RELATED DISORDERS

Prevalence, familial pattern	In the United States, up to 90% of individuals hospitalized for medical care or surgery receive orders for this class of medication during their hospital stay. More that 15% of American adults use these medications, usually by prescription, during any year. Usually a primary care provider prescribes BZs. A 1996 drug survey of use indicated that approximately 6% of individuals acknowledged using either sedatives or tranquilizers illicitly.
Associated descriptive features and mental disorders	Often associated with dependence or abuse with other substances, sometimes sedatives are used to alleviate the unwanted effects of these other substances. Acute intoxication can result in accidental injury from falls and MVAs. Disinheriting effects can lead to aggressive behavior, fights, and legal and interpersonal problems. Severe depressions with suicidal behavior. While there is a wide margin of safety when used alone, benzodiazepines taken in combination with alcohol appear to be particularly dangerous and accidental overdoses have been reported. Tolerance to euphoric effects typically develops quickly while tolerance to brainstem-depressant effects is slower; thus a person taking more substance to achieve euphoria may have a sudden onset of respiratory depression and hypotension, which may result in death. Antisocial behavior and ASPD are associated, especially in those who use illicitly.
Associated laboratory findings	Can be identified in urine and blood. Urine tests are likely to remain positive for up to a week or so after the use of long-acting substances (e.g., flurazepam).
Associated physical examination findings and GMC	On PE, may find a mild decrease in most aspects of ANS functioning (i.e., slower pulse, slightly decreased respiratory rate, slight drop in blood pressure). Consequences of trauma such as internal bleeding or a subdural hematoma may be seen from accidents that occur while intoxicated. IV use of these substances can result in medical complications related to the use of contaminated needles (e.g., hepatitis and HIV).
Course	Typical initial pattern of intermittent use can lead to daily use and high levels of tolerance. With this comes increasing level of interpersonal, work, and legal difficulties as well as increasingly severe episodes of memory impairment, and physiological withdrawal can be expected to ensue. A second, less frequent course begins with an individual who originally obtained the medication by prescription from a physician, usually for the treatment of anxiety, insomnia, or somatic complaints. Tolerance may develop and a substance-seeking pattern unfolds with the person seeking out multiple physicians to obtain supplies of the medication.

(continued)

TABLE 10-37   SEDATIVE-, HYPNOTIC-, OR ANXIOLYTIC-RELATED DISORDERS—
Continued

Differential diagnosis	Primary mental disorders
	Alcohol intoxication
	GMC
	Prior head trauma
	Alcohol withdrawal
	Intoxication with other drugs
	Consequences of physiological conditions (e.g., hyperthyroidism)
	Primary anxiety disorders
	Sedative-, hypnotic-, or anxiolytic-induced disorders
	Note that there are individuals who continue to takes BZ medication according to a physician's direction for a legitimate medication indication over extended periods of time. Even if physiologically dependent on the medication, many of these individuals do not develop symptoms that meet the criteria for dependence because they are not preoccupied with obtaining the substance and its use does not interfere with their performance of usual social or occupational roles.

SOURCE: Adapted from DSM-IV-TR, pp. 284–93.

TABLE 10-38   SPECIFIC CULTURE, AGE, AND GENDER FEATURES OF SEDATIVE-,
HYPNOTIC-, OR ANXIOLYTIC-RELATED DISORDERS

Culture	No specific culture.
Age	Teens and early 20s may illegally obtain to get "high."
	Prescribed use increases with age.
	Elderly have an increased risk for cognitive problems and falls.
Gender	Prescribed use of benzodiazepines is higher in women.

SOURCE: Adapted from DSM-IV-TR, p. 291.

BIBLIOGRAPHY

American Psychiatric Association. *Practice Guidelines for Substance Use Disorders: Alcohol, Cocaine, Opioids.* http://www.psych.org.

Dianostic and Statistical Manual of Mental Disorders, 4th ed., Text Revision (DSM-IV-TR). Washington, DC: American Psychological Association, 2000.

Chapter 11

SCHIZOPHRENIA AND PSYCHOTIC DISORDERS

INTRODUCTION

Psychotic agitated patients are among the most frequent psychiatric emergencies. Determining the cause of the psychosis and agitation is challenging in the emergency situation, where often the patient is not cooperative with giving an accurate history or with other assessment procedures. The clinician must often rely solely on her own experience coupled with collateral contacts/previous records (when available) for emergency assessment.

The question *why now?* is an all-important one in emergency psychiatry and should continually nudge at the clinician in every emergency assessment. For herein lie solution(s). Did the case manager (CM) go on vacation? (Possible solution: The clinician can help set up increased contact with the CM supervisor in the CM's absence. Knowing the likelihood that her patient may decompensate in her absence, the CM may pay special attention in setting up increased contacts with CM supervisor and/or spend more time preparing the patient for her absence.) Was the patient recently discharged from the hospital? (Again there may need to be an increased contact with the mental health agency in this fragile time period.) What is the precipitating stressor to this emergency presentation? A recent move, loss, a medication change, a new medical problem? A conflict with a friend, family member, or neighbor?

There usually is a precipitant, although it may not be of a magnitude that would seem to trigger a crisis. The kindling model of seizure disorder probably best explains this. The summation of stressors builds until finally a seemingly minimal stressor triggers a seizure. Consider that many of the patients who present to psychiatric emergency departments probably have a low threshold for change tolerance so that the slightest or most minimal change may cause them to destabilize. But consider also that these same patients deal with daily environmental stressors that are unimaginable to the average clinician. Most patients presenting to urban psychiatric emergency departments live with poverty, overcrowding, fear of crime, homelessness, unemployment, and poor family support. Environmental factors mingle with complex genetic factors that contribute to their vulnerability to psychotic decompensation. A recent *British Journal of Psychiatry* study (2001) found that the children of poor fathers living in impoverished environments were twice as likely as the children of gainfully employed fathers to grow up to develop schizophrenia.

Often the crisis phase resolves with a supportive, nonjudgmental stance, the readdition of psychotropic medication, and reconnection with case management and community mental health resources. A brief respite in the safety and protection of a crisis stabilization center often fortifies the patient to return to the "front lines" of daily life.

Sometimes, the patient requires hospitalization. Suicide is the leading cause of premature death among patients with schizophrenia; the lifetime incidence of completed suicide among patients with schizophrenia is 10–13%, and an estimated 18–55% of patients with schizophrenia make suicide attempts.

The goals of this chapter include:

1. Review DSM-IV-TR definition of psychosis
2. Review the DSM-IV-TR diagnostic criteria for schizophrenia and subtypes in a clear, concise table format that elucidates prevalence/core symptoms/associated symptoms and comorbidity/course/differential diagnosis
3. Review the DSM-IV-TR diagnostic criteria for psychotic disorders in a clear, concise table format that elucidates prevalence/core symptoms/associated symptoms and comorbidity/course/differential diagnosis
4. Address culture-age-gender considerations for schizophrenia and psychotic disorders in a table format
5. Review emergency biopsychosocial assessment and management

DEFINITIONS

1. Psychosis: Psychosis is historically defined as a loss of ego boundaries or a gross impairment in reality testing. Psychosis as defined in the DSM-IV-TR refers to delusions, prominent hallucinations, disorganized speech, or disorganized or catatonic behavior.
2. Psychotic Disorders: The psychotic disorders include the following:
    Schizophrenia subtypes:
    • Paranoid
    • Catatonic
    • Disorganized

• Undifferentiated
• Residual
    Schizophreniform disorder
    Brief psychotic disorder
    Schizoaffective disorder
    Psychotic disorder NOS
    Psychotic disorder due to a GMC
    Substance-induced psychotic disorder
    Delusional disorder
• Somatic
• Jealous
• Grandiose
• Erotomanic
• NOS
    Shared delusional disorder (formerly folie à deux)
3. Schizophrenia: Schizophrenia involves a constellation of signs and symptoms that impair social and occupational functioning (Tables 11-1 to 11-4).

Characteristic symptoms fall into two categories:

1. Positive symptoms reflect an excess or distortion of normal functioning. These include distortions in the following dimensions:
    • Language (disorganized speech)
    • Thought processes (derailment, incoherence)
    • Thought content (delusions)
    • Perception (hallucinations)
    • Behavior (grossly disorganized or catatonic behavior)
2. Negative symptoms reflect a diminution or loss of normal functions. These include restrictions in the following:
    • Range and intensity of emotional expression (affective flattening)
    • Fluency and productivity of thought and speech (alogia)
    • Initiation of goal-directed behavior (avolition)

Delusions are deemed bizarre if they are clearly implausible, not understandable, and do not derive from ordinary life experiences. If bizarre delusions are present, this single symptom satisfies Criterion 1 for schizophrenia.

TABLE 11-1 DSM-IV-TR SCHIZOPHRENIA

Prevalence and familial pattern	• 0.5–1.5% worldwide. • First-degree biological relatives of individuals with schizophrenia have a risk for schizophrenia that is 10 times greater than that of the general population. • Concordance rates are higher in monozygotic than dizygotic twins.
Core symptoms	A disorder that lasts for at least 6 months and includes at least 1 month of active-phase symptoms (i.e., two or more) of the following: delusions, hallucinations, disorganized speech, disorganized or catatonic behavior, negative symptoms such as alogia, amotivation, poor hygiene.

Subtypes	Core criteria
Paranoid	Preoccupation with one or more delusions or frequent auditory hallucinations. None of the following is prominent: • Disorganized speech • Disorganized or catatonic behavior • Flat or inappropriate affect
Disorganized	Prominent: disorganized speech and disorganized behavior
Catatonic	All of the following are prominent: • Extreme negativism (an apparently motiveless resistance to all instructions or maintenance of a rigid posture against attempts to be moved) or mutism • Peculiarities of voluntary movement as evidenced by posturing (voluntary assumptions of inappropriate or bizarre postures), stereotyped movements, prominent mannerisms, or prominent grimacing • Echolalia or echopraxia
Undifferentiated	Criterion 1 symptoms are present but the criteria are not met for the paranoid, disorganized, or catatonic type
Residual	Absence of prominent delusions, hallucinations, disorganized speech, and grossly disorganized or catatonic behavior Continuing evidence of the disturbance, as indicated by the presence of negative symptoms or two symptoms listed in Criterion 1 for schizophrenia, present in an attenuated form (e.g., odd beliefs, unusual perceptual experiences)

(continued)

TABLE 11-1   DSM-IV-TR SCHIZOPHRENIA—Continued

Associated symptoms/ comorbidity	Estimates of the incidence of concurrent substance abuse or dependency range as high as 40% of persons with schizophrenia, and the lifetime incidence is even higher: 60% in some studies. Substance-related disorders are associated with more frequent and longer periods of hospitalization and other negative outcomes, including homelessness, violence, incarceration, suicide, and HIV infection.
	Anxiety disorders, such as OCD and PD, secondary depression may also be present.
	10% suicide; 20–40% make at least one attempt. In addition to sharing the general risk factors for suicide (see Chapter 7), risk factors for this population include:
	• Recent hospital discharge
	• Post psychotic period
	Lack of insight contributes to poor adherence to medication and higher relapse rates, increased number of involuntary hospital admissions, poorer psychosocial function, and overall poor course of illness.
	Contrary to popular belief, most schizophrenics are not any more dangerous than those in the general population.
Course	Median age of onset for the first psychotic episode is early to mid-20s for men and in the late 20s for women. Typically preceded by a prodromal phase.
	Complete remission (return to full premorbid functioning) is not common. Course is usually variable; some stable, some progressive worsening. The advent of atypical agents has improved the prognosis. Factors associated with a good prognosis include:
	• Good premorbid adjustment
	• Acute onset
	• Later age at onset
	• Absence of poor insight
	• Being female
	• Precipitating events
	• Associated mood disturbance
	• Treatment with antipsychotic medication soon after the onset on the illness consistent with medication adherence
	• Brief duration of active-phase symptoms
	• Good interepisode functioning
	• Minimal residual symptoms
	• Absence of structural brain abnormalities
	• Normal neurological functioning
	• A family history of mood disorder
	• No family history of schizophrenia
Differential diagnosis	*Psychotic due to a GMC*—There are many GMCs that may cause psychotic symptoms. (See Table 11-10.) History, PE, labs will help to distinguish from a primary psychotic disorder.

(continued)

TABLE 11-1   **DSM-IV-TR SCHIZOPHRENIA—Continued**

Delirium—Clues to distinguish from a primary psychotic disorder include history of abrupt onset, variable intensity of symptoms, the presence of visual illusions, prominent impaired attention, and disorientation specifically to time of day. Remember that in schizophrenia, the psychosis tends to be more florid and bizarre with prominent hallucinations, typically auditory.

Dementia—This is a cognitive disorder. Memory functions, particularly short-term memory, is impaired as well as executive functions. Speech may be disorganized. Age and history help in differentiating from schizophrenia or primary psychotic disorder.

Substance-related disorders such as substance-induced psychotic disorder.

Substance-induced delirium and substance-induced persisting dementia—Whether the psychotic symptoms appear to be exacerbated by the substance and to diminish when it has been discontinued.

Relative severity of psychotic symptoms in relation to the amount and duration of substance use.

Knowledge of the characteristic symptoms produced by specific substance.

Schizoaffective disorder—A mood symptom must be present for a substantial portion of the total duration of the disturbance; delusions or hallucinations must be present for at least 2 weeks in the absence of prominent mood symptoms. Mood symptoms in schizophrenia typically:

- Are brief in relation to the total duration of disturbance
- Occur only in prodromal or residual phases
- Do not meet full criteria for mood episode

Depressive disorder NOS or bipolar disorder NOS—These (rather than a specific depressive disorder or bipolar disorder) may be diagnosed if full criteria for a mood episode are superimposed on schizophrenia and are of particular clinical significance.

Mood disorder with psychotic features—This is difficult since mood symptoms are common during all phases of schizophrenia, but in this disorder, psychotic symptoms occur exclusively during periods of mood disturbance.

Mood disorder with catatonic features—This may be particularly difficult to distinguish from schizophrenia, catatonic type. History and collateral information as well as careful attention to chronology of symptoms, i.e., did mood symptoms precede or follow catatonic symptoms?

Schizophreniform—Duration must be at least 1 month but less than 6 months; does not require a decline in functioning.

Schizophrenia involves the presence of symptoms for at least 6 months.

Brief psychotic disorder—Duration for least 1 day but for less than 1 month.

(continued)

TABLE 11-1   **DSM-IV-TR SCHIZOPHRENIA—Continued**

Delusional disorder:
- Usually nonbizarre delusions
- Absence of other characteristic symptoms of schizophrenia

Psychotic disorder NOS.

Pervasive developmental disorders:
- Share disturbances in language affect and interpersonal related-ness, but usually PDD present from infancy or early childhood.
- Absence of prominent delusions, hallucinations.
- Speech is absent, minimal, more sterotypies and abnormalities of prosody.
- Both can be diagnosed.

Childhood presentations combining disordered speech from a *communication disorder* or disorganized behavior from *ADHD schizotypal, schizoid, or paranoid personality disorder.* Both can be diagnosed. Note premorbid for the preexisting personality disorder on Axis II.

Malingering—Malingering must always be included in the differential diagnosis.

Characteristics of malingered hallucinations:
- Vague or inaudible
- Constant
- Command type
- Unaccompanied by delusions
- Stilted language
- Inability to state coping strategies

Characteristics of malingered delusions:
- Abrupt onset and/or termination
- Eagerness to call attention to the delusion
- Bizarre delusions do not seem to affect individual's behavior
- Unaccompanied by other signs/symptoms of psychosis such as disordered thinking

SOURCE: Adapted from DSM-IV-TR, pp. 297–317.

TABLE 11-2 CULTURE/AGE/GENDER CONSIDERATIONS OF SCHIZOPHRENIA

Culture	See Chapter 1 on cultural formulation. The culturally sensitive clinician will be aware of the following: • Ideas that are considered delusional in one culture (e.g., sorcery or witchcraft) may be acceptable in another culture. • Hallucinations may be part of the religious experience in some cultures. • Disorganized speech may in fact be a problem of someone of another culture who has difficulty communicating. • Affective differences in emotional expression, eye contact, and body language are likely with various cultures. • Clinicians have overdiagnosed schizophrenia in some ethnic groups, e.g., African-American and Asian-American, due to clinician bias or cultural insensitivity. Be aware. • Presentation, course, and outcome may all vary according to differences in culture (e.g., catatonic behavior is uncommon in the United States, but common in developing countries). • Individuals in developing countries also tend to have a more acute course and a better outcome than those in industrialized countries.
Age	• Onset is typically in late teens and mid-30s. • In children, delusions and hallucinations may be less elaborated than those observed in adults; visual hallucinations may be more common. • Before diagnosing schizophrenia in children, consider other more common causes of disorganized speech and disorganized behavior, e.g., PDD, communications disorder, ADHD. • Onset can occur after age 45. • Late onset more likely in women than in men. • Persecutory delusions and hallucinations with preservation of affect and social functioning is characteristic.
Gender	Modal age at onset for men is between 18 and 25 years; for women, 25 and mid-30s. 3–10% of women have an age of onset after 40, with better premorbid functioning in women. Women with schizophrenia also tend to have more affective symptomaltology, paranoid delusions, and hallucinations. Men tend to express more negative symptoms. Women have a better prognosis (in short to medium outcome) than men as defined by: • Number of rehospitalizations and lengths of hospital stay • Overall duration of illness • Time to relapse • Response to neuroleptics • Social and work functioning Long-term outcomes for men and women are about the same. Rates of schizophrenia among family members of women with schizophrenia are higher than those among family members of men with schizophrenia, while relatives of men have a higher incidence of schizotypal and schizoid personality traits than do those of women.

SOURCE: Adapted from DSM-IV-TR, pp. 306–8.

TABLE 11-3   **DSM-IV-TR SCHIZOAFFECTIVE DISORDER**

Prevalence/familial pattern	• Less common than schizophrenia. • Increased risk for schizophrenia in first-degree biological relatives of individuals with schizoaffective disorder. • Relatives of individuals with schizoaffective disorder are at increased risk for mood disorders.
Core symptoms	A mood episode and the active-phase symptoms of schizophrenia occur together and were preceded or are followed by at least 2 weeks of delusions of hallucinations without prominent mood symptoms. Two subtypes: bipolar and depressive.
Associated symptoms/ comorbidity	Increased risk for developing pure mood disorders or schizophrenia. Substance-related disorders. Residual symptoms and negative symptoms usually less severe and less chronic that in schizophrenia.
Course	• Early adulthood is typical age of onset. • Substantial occupational and social dysfunction. • Prognosis is better than the prognosis for schizophrenia but worse than the prognosis for mood disorders. • Better prognosis is associated with precipitating stressors and bipolar subtype.
Differential diagnosis	Psychotic disorder due to a GMC Substance-induced psychotic disorder Substance-induced delirium Schizophrenia Mood disorder with psychotic features Delusional disorder Psychotic disorder NOS

SOURCE: Adapted from DSM-IV-TR, pp. 319–23.

TABLE 11-4   **CULTURE/AGE/GENDER FEATURES OF SCHIZOAFFECTIVE DISORDER**

Culture	See Table 11-1.
Age	Schizoaffective disorder, bipolar type, may be more common in young adults. Schizoaffective disorder, depressive type, may be more common in older adults.
Gender	Incidence of schizoaffective disorder is higher in women than in men with an increased incidence among women of the depressive subtype.

SOURCE: Adapted from DSM-IV-TR, p. 321.

TABLE 11-5   **DSM-IV-TR DELUSIONAL DISORDER**

Prevalence	Estimate is 0.03%	
Core symptoms	Presence of one or more nonbizarre delusions that persist for at least 1 month	
	Subtypes	**Central theme**
	Erotomanic	Another person, usually of a higher status, is in love with the individual.
	Grandiose	Conviction of having some great but unrecognized talent or insight or having made some important discovery; having a special relationship with a prominent person or being a prominent person; may have a religious content.
	Jealous	One's partner or spouse is being unfaithful to the individual.
	Persecutory	Person's belief that he or she is being conspired against, cheated, spied on, followed, poisoned or drugged, maliciously maligned, etc.
	Somatic	Involves bodily functions or sensations (e.g., conviction that one emits a foul odor from the skin, mouth, rectum; infestation of insects on or in the skin; an internal parasite; certain body parts are misshapen or ugly; parts of the body are not functioning).
	Mixed	Presence of more than one delusional theme.
	Unspecified	Dominant delusional belief cannot be clearly determined or is not described in the specific types.
Associated symptoms/ comorbidity	• Social, marital, and work problems can result. • Especially with persecutory and jealous subtypes, anger and violence can result, litigious behavior, writing hundreds of letters of protest to judicial officials, court appearances. • MDD, OCD, BDD, and paranoid, schizoid, or avoidant personality disorders may be associated.	
Course	• Hearing deficiency, severe psychosocial stressors such as immigration, and low socioeconomic status may predispose to development of delusional disorder. • Variable onset from adolescence to late in life. • The persecutory type is most common; may be chronic, intermittent.	

(continued)

TABLE 11-5   DSM-IV-TR DELUSIONAL DISORDER—Continued

Differential diagnosis	Delirium, dementia, psychotic disorder due to a GMC
	Substance-induced psychotic disorder
	Schizophrenia
	Schizophreniform disorder
	Mood disorders with psychotic features—If delusions occur exclusively during mood episodes; depressive symptoms are usually mild in delusional disorder, remit while the delusional symptoms persist.
	Psychotic Disorder NOS
	Depressive disorder NOS
	Bipolar disorder NOS
	Shared psychotic disorder
	Brief psychotic disorder
	Psychotic disorder NOS
	Hypochondriasis—Fears of having a serious disease or the concern that one has such a serious disease are held with less than delusional intensity; i.e., the individual can entertain the possibility that the feared disease is not present.
	Body dysmorphic disorder—Preoccupation with some imagined defect in appearance. Beliefs are held with less than delusional intensity and those afflicted may recognize that their view of their appearance is distorted. But criteria for both may be met and both may then be diagnosed: i.e., BDD and delusional disorder, somatic type.
	OCD—Boundary between delusional disorder and OCD especially with poor insight may be hard to establish. If obsessions develop into sustained delusional beliefs that represent a major part of the clinical picture, an additional diagnosis of delusional disorder may be warranted.
	Paranoid Personality Disorder

SOURCE: Adapted from DSM-IV-TR, pp. 323–29.

TABLE 11-6   **CULTURE AND GENDER FEATURES OF DELUSIONAL DISORDER**

Culture	See Table 11-1.
	Consider the particular culture's culturally sanctioned beliefs and delusions that may be culture-specific.
Gender	Jealous subtype is more common in men than in women; otherwise no major gender differences in the overall frequency of delusional disorder.

SOURCE: Adapted from DSM-IV-TR, p. 326.

DSM-IV-TR BRIEF PSYCHOTIC DISORDER (TABLE 11-7)

TABLE 11-7 **DSM-IV-TR BRIEF PSYCHOTIC DISORDER**

Prevalence	Rarely seen in clinical settings in the United States.
Core symptoms	Disturbance that involves the sudden onset of at least one of the following: delusions, hallucinations, disorganized speech, or grossly disorganized or catatonic behavior. Lasts at least 1 day but less than 1 month. Specifiers: • With marked stressor • Without marked stressor • With postpartum onset
Associated symptoms/ comorbidity	Emotional turmoil, overwhelming confusion with severe impairment requiring supervision to attend to basic needs and to provide protection. Increased risk of mortality with a high risk of suicide.
Course	Preexisting personality disorders may predispose to the development of this disorder. Average age at onset is late 20s to early 30s. By definition requires a full remission of all symptoms and a return to premorbid level of functioning within 1 month of the onset of the disturbance.
Differential diagnosis	Psychotic disorder due to a GMC Delirium Substance-induced psychotic disorder Substance-induced delirium Substance intoxication Mood episode Schizophreniform Delusional disorder Mood disorder with psychotic features Psychotic disorder not otherwise specified *Factitious disorder with predominantly psychological signs and symptoms*—Evidence that the symptoms are intentionally produced to assume the patient role. *Malingering*—evidence that the symptoms are feigned for an understandable goal. *Personality disorders*—e.g., BPD psychosocial stressors may precipitate brief periods of psychotic symptoms. Usually transient and do not warrant a separate diagnosis. Only if the psychotic symptoms persist for at least 1 day, an additional diagnosis of brief psychotic disorder may be warranted.

(continued)

TABLE 11-7   DSM-IV-TR BRIEF PSYCHOTIC DISORDER—Continued

Cultural features of brief psychotic disorder	See related schizophrenia table above. Again it is important to distinguish symptoms of brief psychotic disorder from culturally sanctioned response patterns, e.g., hearing voices during a religious ceremony.

SOURCE: Adapted from DSM-IV-TR, pp. 329–32.

DSM-IV-TR SHARED PSYCHOTIC DISORDER (TABLE 11-8)

TABLE 11-8   DSM-IV-TR SHARED PSYCHOTIC DISORDER (FOLIE À DEUX)

Prevalence	Unknown; may get missed.
Core symptoms	Delusions develop in an individual who is involved in a close relationship with another person, sometimes termed the inducer, or the primary case that already has a psychotic disorder with prominent delusions.
Associated symptoms/ comorbidity	Aside from the delusions, behavior is usually not odd or unusual. Impairment is less severe than in the primary case.
Course	Variable, usually chronic, without intervention since typically occurs in relationships that are long-standing and resistant to change.
Differential diagnosis	Schizophrenia Delusional disorder Schizoaffective disorder Mood disorder with psychotic features

SOURCE: Adapted from DSM-IV-TR, pp. 332–34.

DSM-IV-TR PSYCHOTIC DISORDER DUE TO A GENERAL MEDICAL CONDITION (TABLE 11-9)

TABLE 11-9 **DSM-IV-TR PSYCHOTIC DISORDER DUE TO A GENERAL MEDICAL CONDITION**

Prevalence/familial pattern	Underdiagnosed psychotic symptoms may be present in as many as 20% of individuals presenting with untreated endocrine disorders, 15% of SLE patients, and up to 40% of individuals with TLE.
Core symptoms	Prominent hallucinations or delusions that are judged to be due to the direct physiological effects of a GMC (evidence from history, physical examination, or laboratory findings). Subtypes: • With delusions • With hallucinations

Associated symptoms/ comorbidity	**GMCs that may cause psychotic symptoms**	
	Neurological conditions	• Neoplasms • Cerebrovascular disease • Huntington's disease • MS • Epilepsy • Auditory or visual nerve injury or impairment • Deafness • Migraine • CNS infections
	Endocrine conditions	• Hyper- and hypothyroidism • Hyper- and hypoparathyroidism • Hyper- and hypoadrenocortisolism
	Metabolic conditions:	• Hypoxia • Hypercarbia • Hypoglycemia • Fluid or electrolyte imbalances
	Hepatic or renal diseases	• Cirrhosis • Hepatitis • ESRD
	Autoimmune disorders with CNS involvement	Systemic lupus erythematosus

Course	Single transient state or recurrent; treatment may resolve psychotic symptoms but such symptoms may persist even after treatment.

(continued)

Differential diagnosis	Delirium
	Dementia
	Substance-induced psychotic disorder
	Primary psychotic disorder
	Primary mood disorder with psychotic features
	Psychotic disorder NOS

SOURCE: Adapted from DSM-IV-TR, pp. 334–38.

DSM-IV-TR SUBSTANCE-INDUCED PSYCHOTIC DISORDER (TABLE 11-10)

TABLE 11-10   DSM-IV-TR SUBSTANCE-INDUCED PSYCHOTIC DISORDER

Core symptoms	Prominent hallucinations or delusions that are judged to be the direct physiological effects of a substance (drug of abuse, medication, or toxin exposure).

Subtypes:

- With delusions
- With hallucinations

Specifiers:

- *With onset during intoxication*—alcohol, amphetamines and related substances, cannabis, cocaine, hallucinogens, inhalants, opioids, phencyclidine and related drugs, sedatives, hypnotics, anxiolytics, and other or unknown.
- *With onset during withdrawal*—alcohol, sedatives, hypnotics and anxiolytics, and other or unknown substances.

Medications that can evoke psychotic symptoms include:

- Anesthetics and analgesics
- Anticholinergic agents
- Anticonvulsants
- Antidepressants
- Antihistamines
- Antihypertensive agents
- Cardiovascular medications
- Antimicrobial medications
- Antiparkinsonian medications
- Chemotherapeutic agents
- Corticosteroids
- Disulfiram
- Gastrointestinal medications
- Muscle relaxants
- NSAIDS
- Toxins that induce psychotic symptoms:
- Anticholinesterase
- Organophosphate insecticides
- Nerve gases
- Carbon monoxide
- Carbon dioxide
- Volatile substances such as fuel or paint
- OTC meds

Differential diagnosis	*Substance intoxication or substance withdrawal*—Substance-induced psychotic disorder is diagnosed only when the psychotic symptoms are in excess of what you would expect to see with either intoxication or withdrawal and are severe enough to warrant independent clinical attention.
	Hallucinogen persisting perception disorder
	Primary psychotic disorder
	Psychotic disorder due to a GMC
	Psychotic disorder NOS

SOURCE: Adapted from DSM-IV-TR, pp. 338–43.

DSM-IV-TR PSYCHOTIC DISORDER NOS

This category includes:

- Psychotic symptomatology about which there is inadequate information to make a specific diagnosis
- Contradictory information
- Psychosis does not meet criteria for any specific psychotic disorder

Examples include:

- Postpartum psychosis that does not meet criteria for mood disorder with psychotic features, brief psychotic disorder, psychotic disorder due to a GMC- or substance-induced psychotic disorder
- Psychotic symptoms that have lasted for less than 1 month but that have not yet remitted so that the criteria for brief psychotic disorder are not met
- Persistent auditory hallucinations in the absence of any other features
- Persistent nonbizarre delusions with periods of overlapping mood episodes that have been present for a substantial portion of the delusional disturbance
- Situations in which the clinician has concluded that a psychotic disorder is present, but is unable to determine whether it is primary, due to a GMC, or substance-induced

A word on the use of psychotic disorder NOS. There is some controversy regarding the use of this diagnosis in the emergency setting. Some clinicians view this diagnosis as leading to a nonspecific treatment approach. In the authors' view, this is a judicious diagnostic category in the emergency phase. There is a general management approach to the presentation of a psychotic agitated individual such that this diagnosis does not preclude a reasonable clinical management of the patient while a thorough diagnostic assessment is in progress.

EMERGENCY ASSESSMENT AND MANAGEMENT OF SCHIZOPHRENIA AND OTHER PSYCHOTIC DISORDERS (TABLE 11-11)

1. Goals of acute management are:
   a. Maintain safety of patient and the immediate environment
   b. Rapid control of agitation and return to baseline level of functioning
   c. Therapeutic alliance with patient and family
   d. Disposition
2. First break vs. psychotic decompensation in a chronic psychotic disorder

   The goals are essentially the same in both of these situations. However, the first break is even more frightening to the patient and his/her family, since it is more uncertain what the etiology is in a first-break patient, i.e., is the psychosis schizophreniform, schizophrenia, substance-induced, and/or a GMC? As the risk of an untoward side effect from antipsychotic medication is high; it is best to hospitalize a first-break patient.

TABLE 11-11   **SUMMARY OF BIOPSYCHOSOCIAL ASSESSMENT MANAGEMENT**

Biological

Assessment

• Psychiatric and general medical history • Brief focused physical and neurological examinations • Mental status exam • Collateral interviews	Labs may include: • Drug screen-urine tox • CBC/electrolytes/renal function/liver function • Thyroid function • ECG if history of cardiovascular disease

Assessment would also include suicide risk and violent risk assessment.

Management

Medications	• Conventional vs. atypical—see Chapter 3 for specific medications and dosages • Choosing medication: consider past history of medication response • Side effect profile • Drug-drug-interactions • Patient preference • Intended route of administration • PO vs. IM: Choosing a dose that maximizes benefit and minimizes uncomfortable side effects is the ideal. 2–20 mg haloperidol or 300–1000 mg chlorpromazine, 4–6 mg risperiodone, 10–20 mg olanzapine, 20–24 mg sertindole. • Benzodiazepines such as lorazepam are often added to the antipsychotic to help reduce agitation and anxiety associated with psychotic symptoms. The combination of lorazepam and high-potency antipsychotic medication has been found to be safer and more effective than large doses of antipsychotic medication in controlling excitement and motor agitation.

(continued)

	Management	
	SE Management	Anti-EPS medications such as cogentin and diphenhydramine may be given prophylactically if the patient prefers it and has a history of EPS.
Psychosocial	• Quiet environment • Supportive stance • Education • Encouragement • Explanations • Expectations	

BIBLIOGRAPHY

American Psychiatric Association. *Practice Guidelines for the Treatment of Schizophrenia.* http://www.psych.org.

British Journal of Psychiatry (October 2001).

Caldwell CB, Gottesman II. Schizophrenics Kill Themselves Too: A Review of Risk Factors for Suicide. *Schizophrenia Bulletin* 16(4) (1990): 571–89.

Diagnostic and Statistical Manual of Mental Disorders, 4th ed., Text Revision (DSM-IV-TR). Washington, DC: American Psychiatric Association, 2000.

Forster P, et al. Phenomenology and Treatment of Psychotic Disorders in the Psychiatric Emergency Service. *Psychiatric Clinics of North America* 22(4) (1999): 735–55.

Resnick PJ. *Malingering Principles and Practice of Forensic Psychiatry*, ed. Rosner, R New York: Oxford University Press, 1998.

Chapter 12

PERSONALITY DISORDERS

INTRODUCTION

Over 90% of patients with Axis II personality disorders have one or more Axis I disorders (DSM-IV-TR, 2000). Since Axis II often underlies Axis I presentations, it is important to understand the three clusters of personality disorders and how they may color the individual patient's presentation. While the authors will provide the DSM-IV-TR criteria of each of the personality disorders, we agree with Weston (1997) regarding how clinicians *really* diagnose personality disorders. Rather than asking about specific criteria (e.g., "Do you have a history of lying, cheating, recklessness, and in general total disregard for the feelings of others?" for antisocial personality disorder [ASPD] or "Do you have a history of being emotionally shallow, suggestible, naïve, uncomfortable not being the center of attention?" for histrionic personality disorder [HPD]), clinicians form clinical impressions of personality traits while interviewing a patient, listening to the way the patient presents his story, and observing his mental status and his demeanor with family, staff, and the clinician.

Clinicians are also influenced by the medical record and by psychological testing available (Othmer and Othmer 2001). The authors advise that assuming the presence of a personality disorder until proven otherwise is clinically wise. When working with patients in crisis, personality disorder, along with general medical conditions, substance-use disorders, malingering, and factitious disorders, must all be in the forefront in the differential diagnoses.

The goals of this chapter include:

1. Review DSM-IV-TR general diagnostic criteria for personality disorders
2. Review in table format the DSM-IV-TR diagnostic criteria of each personality disorder (PD) and dissociative identity disorder (formerly multiple personality disorder), including: prevalence/familial pattern, core symptoms, associated symptoms/comorbidity, and differential diagnosis
3. Review in table format the culture/age/gender features unique to personality disorders
4. Review general biopsychosocial emergency management guidelines for personality disorders; also review guidelines specific to each disorder

DSM-IV-TR DEFINTIONS

1. Personality traits are enduring patterns of perceiving, relating to, and thinking about the environment and oneself that are exhibited in a wide range of social and personal contexts.
2. Personality disorder is an enduring pattern of inner experience and behavior that deviates markedly from the expectations of the individual's culture, is pervasive and inflexible, has an onset in adolescence or early adulthood, is stable over time, and leads to distress or impairment.

   Typically it manifests in dysfunction in the following areas:
   - Cognition (i.e., ways of perceiving and interpreting self, other people, and events)
   - Affectivity (i.e., the range, intensity, lability, and appropriateness of emotional response)
   - Interpersonal functioning
   - Impulse control

While these disorders tend to take shape in childhood and adolescence, they are not diagnosed until young adulthood.

GENERAL GUIDELINES FOR APPROACHING PERSONALITY DISORDERS IN THE EMERGENCY PHASE

1. Expect to see personality disorders as part of the clinical picture. Patients rarely present with chief complaints about their personality disorder. Typically a patient presents with complaints of mood, anxiety, or other Axis I disorder symptoms. But an individual's personality disorder wholly colors his presentation, response to treatment, disposition options, and follow-through.
2. Be professional always. The clinician should be respectful, patient, and firm. She deftly manages the inevitable negative countertransference typically provoked by the personality-disordered.
3. Keep an eye on the prize. The prize in this case is the completion of acute-phase goals: diagnostic clarification, rapid stabilization, and timely disposition. Processing the crisis with the patient is an important part of this process. Briefly reviewing what happened and why, plus reviewing options for future potential triggering situations, can be useful. Avoid confrontation in the emergency phase; it is not necessary or useful to challenge or confront a maladaptive personality style in this phase. Nor does it further acute-phase goals.
4. Be realistic. A clinician should aim for stabilization to a baseline level of function. Emergency psychiatry patients are seldom highly functional, flexible personality styles with healthy defense mechanisms at baseline. Aim for close to baseline.
5. Believe that change is possible. The authors advise framing a hopeful response; i.e., talk about change as possible when reviewing disposition recommendations with the patient.

CLUSTER A

Cluster A PDs are odd, eccentric, and paranoid and include:

Paranoid personality disorder (PPD) (Tables 12-1 to 12-3)

Schizoid personality disorder (schizoid PD) (Tables 12-4 to 12-6)

Schizotypal personality disorder (schizotypal PD) (Tables 12-7 to 12-9)

TABLE 12-1 DSM-IV-TR PARANOID PERSONALITY DISORDER

Prevalence/familial pattern	0.5–2.5% general population 10–30% inpatient psychiatric settings 2–10% outpatient mental health clinics Increased prevalence of paranoid personality disorder in relatives of probands with chronic schizophrenia and for a more specific familial relationship with delusional disorder, persectory type
Core	Pattern of distrust and suspiciousness such that others' motives are interpreted as malevolent
Associated symptoms/ comorbidity	Difficult to get along with, problems with close relationships Combative and suspicious nature often elicits hostile responses from others, thus confirming their original expectations Brief psychotic episodes Delusional disorder, MDD, agoraphobia, OCD, substance disorders and co-occurring personality disorders such as schizoptypal, schizoid, narcissistic, avoidant, and borderline
Differential diagnosis	*Delusional disorder, persectory type* *Schizophrenia, paranoid type* *Mood disorder with psychotic features* All are characterized by a period of persistent psychotic symptoms. To qualify for an additional diagnosis of paranoid personality disorder, the personality disorder must have been present before the onset of psychotic symptoms and must persist when the psychotic symptoms are in remission. *Personality change due to a GMC:* Traits emerge due to the direct effects of a GMC *Substance-induced personality change:* Traits emerge due to the direct effects of substances *Paranoid traits associated with the development of physical handicaps, e.g., hearing impairment* *Other Personality Disorders:*

PD	Shared Characteristics	Differentiating Characteristics
Schizoptypal	Suspiciousness	Schizoptypal also include odd beliefs and ideas.
Schizoid PD	Experienced as cold and aloof	Prominent paranoid ideation in PPD.
Borderline and histrionic PD	Show a tendency to react to minor stimuli with anger	Neither BPD nor HPD is typically associated with pervasive suspiciousness.
Avoidant PD	Reluctance to confide in others	APD: due to fear of being embarrassed or found inadequate rather than from fear of others' malicious intent.

(continued)

TABLE 12-1   DSM-IV-TR PARANOID PERSONALITY DISORDER—Continued

PD	Shared Characteristics	Differentiating Characteristics
Antisocial PD	Antisocial behavior	ASPD is motivated by a desire for personal gain or to exploit others; PPD is motivated by a desire for revenge.
Narcissistic PD	Suspiciousness, social withdrawal, or alienation	NPD fears having their imperfections or flaws revealed.

Paranoid traits may be adaptive particulary in threatening environments. Again, it is only when these traits are inflexible, maladaptive, and persisting, and cause significant functional impairment or subjective distress, that a personality disorder should be diagnosed.

SOURCE: Adapted from DSM-IV-TR, pp. 685–729.

TABLE 12-2 CULTURE/AGE/GENDER CONSIDERATIONS OF PARANOID PERSONALITY DISORDER

Culture	Members of minority groups, immigrants, polical and economic refugees, or individuals of different ethnic backgrounds may display guarded or defensive behaviors due to unfamiliarity (language barriers or lack of knowledge of rules and regulations) or in response to the perceived neglect or indifference of the majority society.
Age	• May first become apparent in childhood with solitariness, poor peer relationships, social anxiety, underachievement in school. • Hypersensitivity, peculiar thoughts and language, and idiosyncratic fantasies may also emerge in childhood. • Such children or adolescents may appear odd or eccentric and attract teasing.
Gender	Males are diagnosed more commonly than females in clinical samples.

SOURCE: Adapted from DSM-IV-TR, p. 692.

TABLE 12-3 BIOPSYCHOSOCIAL MANAGEMENT GUIDELINES SPECIFIC TO PARANOID PERSONALITY DISORDER

Biological	Psychotropic medications may be indicated for acute symptoms such as acute psychotic symptoms.
Psychosocial	• Rapport is usually difficult since these patients, by definition, lack trust in others. • Turn off the warmth with these patients, be honest, and concentrate in focusing on the troubles leading to their current presentation. • Be aware that questions will likely be viewed with suspicion. • Get the information that will help make a decision regarding disposition. • Make it known why certain questions are asked and why the answers are relevant to your decision-making process. • There is little evidence-based research into this disorder, since most patients do not present because of their personality disorders (at least not knowingly) but rather because of Axis I disorders or other breakdown in usual coping styles. • Family, group, and self-help interventions have not been found to be effective in this PD.

TABLE 12-4   DSM-IV-TR SCHIZOID PERSONALITY DISORDER

Prevalence/familial pattern	Uncommon in clinical settings.
Core	• Pattern of detachment from social relationships and a restricted range of emotional expression • Increased prevalence in the relatives of individuals with schizophrenia or schizotypal persoality disorder
Associated symptoms/ comorbidity	• Directionless lives, adrift • Lack of social skills and lack of desire for sexual experiences lead to few friendships and no marriage • Can work best under conditions of social isolation • Can experience brief psychotic episodes under stress • May be antecedent to development of delusional disorder or schizophrenia; may be associated with MDD • Co-occurs with schizoptypal, paranoid, and avoidant personality disorders
Differential diagnosis	*Delusional disorder, persecutory type* *Schizophrenia, paranoid type* *MDD disorder with psychotic features* All are characterized by a period of persistent psychotic symptoms. To qualify for an additional diagnosis of paranoid personality disorder, the personality disorder must have been present before the onset of psychotic symptoms and must persist when the psychotic symptoms are in remission. *Autistic disorder and Asperger's disorder*—Milder forms have more severely impaired social interaction and stereotyped behavior and interests. *Personality change due to a GMC*—traits emerge due to the direct effects of a GMC. *Symptoms that develop in association with chronic substance use*—Traits emerge due to the direct effects of substances. *Other Personality Disorders:*

PD	Shared Characteristics	Differentiating Characteristics
Schizotypal PD		The presence of cognitive and perceptual disorders distinguish it from schizoid.
Paranoid PD		The presence of suspiciousness and paranoid ideation distinguish it from schizoid.

(continued)

TABLE 12-4   DSM-IV-TR SCHIZOID PERSONALITY DISORDER—Continued

PD	Shared Characteristics	Differentiating Characteristics
Avoidant PD	Social isolation	Due to fear of being embarrassed or found inadequate and excessive anticipation of rejection rather than the more pervasive detachment and limited desire for social intimacy found in schizoid personality disorder.
Obsessive-compulsive PD	Social detachment	Stemming from devotion to work and discomfort with emotions; do have a capacity for intimacy.

"Loners"—Only when these traits are inflexible and maladaptive and cause significant functional impairment or subjective distress would they be considered a personality disorder.

SOURCE: Adapted from DSM-IV-TR, pp. 694–97.

TABLE 12-5 CULTURE/AGE/GENDER CONSIDERATIONS OF SCHIZOID PERSONALITY DISORDER

Culture	Consider cultural background; immigrants may be perceived as cold, hostile, or indifferent. Consider whether the individual has recently moved from rural to urban area, which may result in a period of "emotional freezing."
Age	May first become apparent in childhood or adolescence; manifest with solitariness, poor peer relationships, and underachievement in school; marks these children as different and may lead to teasing.
Gender	Diagnosed slightly more often in males than in females.

SOURCE: Adapted from DSM-IV-TR, pp. 695–96.

TABLE 12-6 BIOPSYCHOSOCIAL MANAGEMENT GUIDELINES SPECIFIC TO SCHIZOID PERSONALITY DISORDER

Biological	Acute symptom relief; Axis I disorders
Psychosocial	• Treatment of choice for this as well as most of the personality disorders is individual long-term psychotherapy. • In the acute phase. • Be aware that trust and rapport may be difficult. • Spell out the goals of your intervention clearly, focus on simple treatment goals. • Outpatient individual therapy is best. • Family, couples. • Self-help—if supportive, nonintrusive group can supplement individual.

TABLE 12-7 DSM-IV-TR SCHIZOTYPAL PERSONALITY DISORDER

Prevalence/familial pattern	• 3% of general population • Appears to aggregate familialy • More prevalent among the first-degree biological relatives of individuals with schizophrenia than among the general population • Modest increase in schizophrneia and other psychotic disorders in the relatives of probands with schizoptypal personality disorder
Core	Pattern of acute discomfort in close relationships, cognitive or perceptual distortions, and eccentricities of behavior
Associated symptoms/ comorbidity	• Under stress, may experience transient psychotic episodes occasionally becoming clinically significant enough to warrant an additional diagnosis of an Axis I psychotic disorder • 30–50% with this diagnosis also have a concurrent diagnosis of MDD when admitted to a clinical setting • Also co-occurrence with schizoid, paranoid, avoidant, and borderline personality disorders
Differential diagnosis	*Delsuional disorder* *Schizophrenia* *Mood disorder with psychotic features* All are characterized by a period of persistent psychotic symptoms. An additional diagnosis of schizotypal personality disorder can be made only if the symptoms preceded the onset of psychotic symptoms and persist when the psychotic symptoms are in remission. *Austistic disorder, Asperger's disorder* *Expressive and mixed receptive-expressive language disorder* *Communcication disorders* Solitary odd children whose behavior is characterized by marked social isolation, eccentricity, or peculiarities of language may be differentiated by the primacy and severity of the disorder in language accompanied by compensatory efforts by the child to communicate by other means (e.g., gestures and by the characteristic features of impaired language found in a specialized language assessment). Milder forms of *autistic disorder and Asperger's disorder* are differentiated by the even greater lack of social awareness and emotional reciprocity and stereotyped behaviors and interests. *Personality change due to GMC:* Traits emerge due to the direct effects of a GMC. *Symptoms that develop in association with chronic substance use:* Traits emerge due to the direct effects of substances. *Other Personality Disorders:*

PD	Shared Characteristics	Differentiating Characteristics
Paranoid	Social detachment	Lack of suspiciousness and paranoid in Schizotypal
Avoidant	Lack of close relationships	More pervasive detachment and limited desire from social intimacy in Schizotypal.

(continued)

TABLE 12-7   **DSM-IV-TR SCHIZOTYPAL PERSONALITY DISORDER—Continued**

PD	Shared Characteristics	Differentiating Characteristics
Narcissistic	Display suspiciousness, social withdrawal or alienation	In NPD fear having flaws revealed
Borderline	Transient psychotic-like symptoms Social isolation	Are usually more closely related to affective shifts in response to stress (e.g., intense anger, anxiety, or disappointment) and are usually more dissociative (e.g., derealization or depersonalization). In contrast, individuals with schizoptypal PD have more enduring psychotic-like symptoms that may worsen under stress, are not typically associated with affective shifts. Social isolation in BPD is typically secondary to repeated interpersonal failures due to angry outbursts and frequent mood shifts rather than a result of a persistent lack of social contacts and desire for intimacy. BPD is also usually associated with impulsive or manipulative behaviors. But there is a high rate of co-occurrence between schizotypal and BPD.

Schizotypal features during adolescence may be less a reflection of enduring personality disorder and more a reflection of transient emotional turmoil sometimes associated with adolescence.

SOURCE: Adapted from DSM-IV-TR, pp. 697–701.

TABLE 12-8 CULTURE/AGE/GENDER CONSIDERATIONS OF SCHIZOTYPAL PERSONALITY DISORDER

Culture	Pervasive culturally determined characteristics such as those regarding religious beliefs and rituals may appear schizotypal (e.g., voodoo, speaking in tongues, life beyond death, shamanism, mind reading, sixth sense, evil eye, magical beliefs related to health and illness).
Age	May first become apparent in childhood and adolescence with solitariness, poor peer relationships, social anxiety, underachievement in school, hypersensitivity, peculiar thoughts and language, and bizarre fantasies. Such children may appear odd or eccentric and attract teasing from peers.
Gender	Slightly more common in males than females.

SOURCE: Adapted from DSM-IV-TR, p. 699.

TABLE 12-9 BIOPSYCHOSOCIAL MANAGEMENT GUIDELINES SPECIFIC TO SCHIZOTYPAL PERSONALITY DISORDER

Biological	Medications in acute psychotic symptoms
Psychosocial	• Long-term individual psychotherapy is the ultimate treatment of choice.
	In the emergency phase:
	• Do not directly challenge delusional inappropriate thoughts.
	• Supportive.
	Non-emergency-phase treatment:
	• Social skills training.
	• Group that is specific to this disorder as progress is made in individual therapy.
	• Self-help is unhelpful and possibly harmful.

CLUSTER B

Cluster B PDs are erratic and dramatic and include:

Antisocial personality disorder (ASPD) (Tables 12-10 to 12-12)

Borderline personality disorder (BPD) (Tables 12-13 to 12-15)

Histrionic personality disorder (HPD) (Tables 12-16 to 12-18)

Narcissitic personality disorder (NPD) (Tables 12-19 to 12-21)

TABLE 12-10 DSM-IV-TR ANTISOCIAL PERSONALITY DISORDER

Prevalence/familial pattern	• 3% in males and 1% in females in general population • 3–30% in clinical population, higher in substance abuse treatment settings and prison or forensic settings • More common among the first-degree biological relatives of those with the disorder than among the general population • The risk to biological relatives of females with this disorder higher than the risk of biological relatives to males with this disorder • In families that have a member with ASPD, males more often have ASPD and females more often have somatization disorder • Adoption studies show that both genetic and environmental factors contribute to the risk of this group of disorders • Both adopted and biological children of parents with ASPD have an increased risk of developing ASPD, somatization disorder, and substance-related disorders • Adopted-away children resemble their biological parents more than their adoptive parents although the adoptive family environment influences the risk of developing a personality disorder
Core	Pattern of willful disregard of, and violation of, the rights of others
Associated symptoms/ comorbidity	• Lack empathy • Callous, cynical, and contemptuous of the feelings, rights, and sufferings of others • Inflated and arrogant self-appraisal • Excessively opinionated, self-assured, or cocky • Glib, superficial charm • Voluble, verbal facility • Irresponsible and exploitative in their sexual relationships • Irresponsible parents • More likely to die by violent means • May also experience dysphoria with complaints of tension, inability to tolerate boredom, depressed mood • Associated anxiety disorders, depressive disorders, substance-related disorders, somatization disorder, pathological gambling, and other disorders of impulse control may co-occur • May also have co-occurring BPD, and NPD features or disorders. • Increased likelihood of developing ASPD if individual has early-onset conduct disorder (before age 10) and ADHD

(continued)

TABLE 12-10 **DSM-IV-TR ANTISOCIAL PERSONALITY DISORDER—Continued**

	Child abuse or neglect, unstable or erratic parenting, or inconsistent parental discipline may increase the likelihood that conduct disorder will evolve into ASPD.
Differential diagnosis	Not given to individuals under age 18 and only if there is a history of some symptoms of conduct disorder before age 15 *Substance-related disorders* *Schizophrenia* *Manic episode* *Other Personality Disorders:*

Disorder	Shared Characteristics	Differentiating Characteristics
NPD	Tendency to be glib, tough-minded, superficial	NPD usually lacks the history of conduct disorder in childhood or criminal behavior in adulthood Need admiration and envy of others
HPD	Tendency to be impulsive, superficial, excitement seeking, reckless, seductive, and manipulative	More exaggerated in emotions Do not tend to engage in antisocial behaviors
BPD	Manipulative	Manipulative to gain nurturance rather than to gain power, profit, or material gratification More emotionally unstable and less aggressive than ASPD
PPD	May share antisocial behavior	PPD: Antisocial behavior is motivated by a desire for revenge rather than a desire for personal gain or to exploit others

	Adult antisocial behavior—Criminal, aggressive, or other antisocial behavior that comes to clinical attention but that does not meet the full criteria for ASPD. Only when antisocial personality traits are inflexible, maladaptive, and persistent and cause significant functional impairment or subjective distress do they constitute ASPD.

Source: Adapted from DSM-IV-TR, pp. 701–6.

TABLE 12-11   CULTURE/AGE/GENDER CONSIDERATIONS OF ANTISOCIAL PERSONALITY DISORDER

Culture	Associated with low socioeconomic status and urban settings. Consider the social and economic context in which the antisocial behaviors occur (i.e., is the antisocial behavior part of a protective survival strategy?).
Age	By definition, not diagnosed before age 18 years.
Gender	Much more common in males than females but could be underdiagnosed in females. Note what we have learned about the capacity of females to be extremely aggressive and violent.

SOURCE: Adapted from DSM-IV-TR, pp. 703–4.

TABLE 12-12   BIOPSYCHOSOCIAL MANAGEMENT GUIDELINES SPECIFIC TO ANTISOCIAL PERSONALITY DISORDER

Biological	Psychotropics for acute symptoms and for diagnosed Axis I disorders
Psychosocial	• Long-term individual psychotherapy • Group-structured • Family, couples • Self-help

TABLE 12-13 **DSM-IV-TR BORDERLINE PERSONALITY DISORDER**

Prevalence/familial pattern	• 2% in general population • 10% in outpatient mental health clinics • 20% among psychiatric inpatients • 30–60% among clinical populations with personality disorders • About five times more common among the first-degree biological relatives of those with the disorder than in the general population • Increased familial risk for substance-related disorders, ASPD, and mood disorders
Core	Pattern of instability in interpersonal relationships, self-image, and affects, and marked impulsivity

Associated symptoms/ comorbidity	• Pattern of undermining themselves at the moment a goal is about to be realized (e.g., dropping out of school just before graduation, regressing severely after a discussion of how well therapy is going, destroying a good relationship just when it is clear that the relationship could last)
	• Psychotic-like symptoms during times of stress
	• May feel more secure with transitional objects (e.g., a pet or inanimate possession) than in interpersonal relationships
	• Premature death from suicide
	• Especially in those with co-occurring mood disorders or substance-related disorders
	• Physical handicaps from self-inflicted abuse behaviors or failed suidicide attempts
	• Recurrent job losses
	• Interrupted education
	• Broken marriages
	• Physical and sexual abuse, neglect, hostile conflict, early parental loss or separation is more common in the childhood histories of those with BPD.
	• Commonly co-occurring Axis disorders:
	  • Mood disorders
	  • Substance-related disorders
	  • Eating disorders
	  • PTSD
	  • ADHD
	  • Other personality disorders

Differential diagnosis	*Mood disorders:* Often co-occurs. Be aware that the cross-sectional presentation of BPD can be mimicked by an episode of mood disorder, so avoid giving an additional diagnosis of BPD without having documented the pattern of behavior. Has an early onset and a long-standing course.

(continued)

TABLE 12-13   DSM-IV-TR BORDERLINE PERSONALITY DISORDER—Continued

Other Personality Disorders:

PD	Shared Characteristics	Differentiating Characteristics
HPD	Attention-seeking Manipulative behavior Rapidly shifting emotions	Self-destructiveness Angry disruptions in close relation-ships Chronic feelings of deep emptiness and loneliness
Schizotypal PD	Paranoid ideas or illusions	Paranoid ideas are more transient in BPD, more interpersonally reactive, and responsive to external structuring
Paranoid PD and NPD	Angry reaction to minor stimuli	PPD and NPD have relative stability of self-image, relative lack of self-destructiveness, impulsivity, and abandonment concerns
ASPD	Manipulative behavior	ASPD manipulates to gain profit, power, or some other material gain while BPD manipulates to gain the concern of caretakers.
Dependent PD	Fear of abandonment	BPD reacts to abandonment with feelings of emotional emptiness, rage, and demands, whereas the DPD reacts with increasing appeasement and submissiveness and urgently seeks a replacement relationship to provide caregiving and support. BPD also typically has a pattern of unsta-ble and intense relationships

Personality change due to a GMC—Traits emerge due to the direct effects of a GMC.

Symptoms that may develop in association with chronic substance use—Traits emerge due to the direct effects of substances.

Identity problem—reserved for identity concerns related to a developmental phase and does not qualify as a mental disorder.

SOURCE: Adapted from DSM-IV-TR, pp. 706–10.

TABLE 12-14   CULTURE/AGE/GENDER CONSIDERATIONS OF BORDERLINE PERSONALITY DISORDER

Culture	Found in many settings and cultures worldwide
Age	Adolescents and young adults with identity problems may transiently display behaviors that may mistakenly give the impression of BPD. But consider the situational stressors that may occur at this time of life—anxiety-provoking choices, conflicts about sexual orientation, competing social pressures to decide on careers, and other existential dilemmas—before making a diagnosis of BPD.
Gender	75% females

SOURCE: Adapted from DSM-IV-TR, p. 708.

TABLE 12-15 BIOPSYCHOSOCIAL MANAGEMENT GUIDELINES SPECIFIC TO BORDERLINE PERSONALITY DISORDER

Biological	Psychotropic medication use is controversial in this disorder. Since many of the mood states are temporary, it is questionable how valuable it is to treat with medications. On the other hand, medications may help to reduce the frequency and severity of mood lability and temporary psychotic episodes. It is best to avoid polypharmacy in this population due to the risk of suicide by overdose, and/or to choose medications in part on the basis of their safety profile in overdose. Axis I disorders, if diagnosed, should be treated with the appropriate medication but do avoid chasing after symptoms, which may be more due to the PD than attributable to an Axis I disorder.
Psychosocial	In the acute phase, it is best to be firm in approach. Be aware that such patients operate with a primitive defense style that includes splitting, manipulation, and devaluing/idealizing.
	If there is a case manager and/or primary treater, contact them immediately to help with the crisis and problem solving and to improve a consolidated treatment stance. Remember the splitting? Avoid it by communicating with caregivers. It is not always possible, but document that you tried and what you were trying to accomplish.
	Hospitalize if the patient threatens to commit suicide should she be discharged. The authors see little point in struggling over this. A brief restabilizing admission usually stabilizes the patient. If the patient insists she is suicidal, it is the authors' experience that trying to change her mind is an exasperating waste of time.
	Projective identification is a defense mechanism that works as follows: BPD patient experiences an unacceptable emotion (rage) and projects this onto clinician. Clinician, otherwise calm and serene, feels a surge of anger in the presence of BPD patient. Clinician then behaves with an angry demeanor toward BPD, to which BPD reacts angrily and, in her mind, justifiably. It is a bewildering experience but it should take a wise clinician just a couple of those experiences before he mentally prepares to be in the presence of the BPD patient.
	Thus, preparation is important: a calm, firm frame of mind, limit setting, firm directives, and expectations voiced clearly (e.g., "I can see you are upset; I want to talk this over with you but we will need to do so in a quiet room so that we do not disturb other patients here who are also struggling with problems. If you cannot calm yourself down, we can offer you medication to help do so."). Make it clear that violence is not acceptable and will be dealt with swiftly resulting in a seclusion or restraint if need be. In effect, the clinician offers his stability in contrast to the patient's lability. These are challenging patients, and they are damaged people, often from repeated abuse in childhood, and are deserving of care.

(continued)

In the nonacute phases of treatment, the best approach to emerge in the late twentieth century is Marsha Linehan's Dialectical Behavioral Therapy (DBT). This is a spin-off of CBT with emphasis on correcting cognitive distortion and emotional regulation. DBT is a restructuring program that has proven via evidence-based designs to be effective in reducing the severity and frequency of acting out in BPD.

Individual, group, family, and couples therapy may all play a role in working with the BPD. In addition, in particularly severe cases, case management may be helpful with a multidisciplinary team.

TABLE 12-16 **DSM-IV-TR HISTRIONIC PERSONALITY DISORDER**

Prevalence/familial pattern	• 2–3% in general population • 10–15% in inpatient and outpatient settings
Core	Pattern of excessive emotionality and attention seeking
Associated symptoms/ comorbidity	• Difficulty achieving intimacy • Difficulty with same-sex friendships • Excessive need to be center of attention and may become depressed if not • Appears "fake," shallow • Craves excitement • Often starts new friendships and activities with enthusiasm but then loses interest • Suicidal gestures and threats may be to get attention and coerce better caregiving. May have associated Axis I disorders such as anxiety disorders, depressive disorders, somatization disorder, and co-occurring personality disorders such as BPD, NPD, ASPD, and dependent PD.
Differential diagnosis	*Other personality disorders:*

PD	Shared Characteristics	Differentiating Characteristics
BPD	Attention seeking Manipulative behavior Rapidly shifting emotions	BPD also includes: Self-destructiveness, angry disruptions in close relationships, chronic feelings of deep emptiness and identity disturbance.
ASPD	Impulsive Superficial Excitement seeking Reckless Seductive Manipulative	ASPD is manipulative to gain profit, power, or some other material gratification; HPD is manipulative to gain nurturance.
NPD	Crave attention; may exaggerate the intimacy of their relationships with others	NPD wants praise for "superiority" whereas HPD is willing to be viewed as fragile or dependent as this will gain attention. NPD emphasizes the "VIP" status or wealth of friends.
DPD	Excessive dependence on others for praise and guidance	HPD is more flamboyant, exaggerated, and emotional than DPD.

Personality change due to a GMC: Traits emerge due to the direct effects of a GMC.

Symptoms that may develop in association with chronic substance use: Histrionic personality traits are exhibited by many individuals; only if these are inflexible, maladaptive, and persisting and cause significant functional impairment or subjective distress do they constitute HPD.

TABLE 12-17   CULTURE/AGE/GENDER CONSIDERATIONS OF HISTRIONIC PERSONALITY DISORDER

Culture	Norms for interpersonal behavior, personal appearance, and emotional expressiveness vary widely across cultures. Consider the various traits (emotionality, seductiveness, dramatic interpersonal style, novelty seeking, sociability, charm, impressionability, and a tendency to somatization) in the context of cultural norms and whether these traits cause clinically significant impairment or distress.
Age	Nonspecific.
Gender	In clinical settings, more often seen in females. Males may be "macho," seeking to be center of attention by bragging about athletic skills. Females may wear very feminine clothes and brag about how much they impressed the dance instructor.

SOURCE: Adapted from DSM-IV-TR, p. 712.

TABLE 12-18   BIOPSYCHOSOCIAL MANAGEMENT GUIDELINES SPECIFIC TO HISTRIONIC PERSONALITY DISORDER

Biological	Identified Axis I disorders and acute symptoms may be treated. Be aware of the impulsive nature of this PD and avoid polypharmacy and unnecessary psychotropic medications.
Psychosocial	Such patients may present in the emergency or crisis situation because of situational factors that overwhelm their already tenuous coping mechanisms. Such patients are, unlike other PDs, more likely to seek treatment quickly and, again, usually in a crisis as a means of coping with their need. Individual therapy is, again, the treatment of choice.
	With these patients, a clinician needs to guard against a "rescuer role"; often the therapist is perceived as sexually attractive to the patient and she behaves in a seductive or helpless manner to be nurtured or rescued by him. Again, preparation will be the best prevention for falling into that particular situation. Setting firm boundaries, making it clear that the therapeutic relationship is just that, therapeutic, and nothing more.
	Solution-focused is probably best.
	Group/family therapy may only reinforce the patient's need to be the center of attention and lead to greatly exaggerating her behaviors.

TABLE 12-19   **DSM-IV-TR NARCISSISTIC PERSONALITY DISORDER**

Prevalence/familial pattern	>1% in general population; 2–16% in clinical population.
Core	Pattern of grandiosity, need for admiration, and lack of empathy.
Associated symptoms/ comorbidity	• Vulnerability in self-esteem leads to sensitivity to injury from criticism or defeat.
	• Criticism haunts them and leaves them feeling humiliated, degraded, hollow, and empty.
	• May react with rage, disdain, defiant counterattack.
	• Humility as mask to protect the grandiosity.
	• Impaired interpersonal relationships due to entitlement, constant need for admiration, and disregard for the sensitivities of others.
	• High achievement due to overweening ambition and confidence or low achievement due to unwillingness to take a risk in competitive or other situations in which defeat is possible.
	• Sustained feelings of shame or humiliation and the attendant self-criticism may be associated with social withdrawal, depressed mood.
	• Dysthymia, MDD, hypomania.
	• Anorexia nervosa, substance-related disorders, and other personality disorders may co-occur.
Differential diagnosis	*Other Personality Disorders:*

PD	Shared Characteristics	Differentiating Characteristics
HPD	Require attention	NPD requires attention and feels excessive pride in achievements
		Relative lack of emotional display
		Disdain for others' sensitivities
ASPD	Tough-minded	NPD is not:
	Glib	Impulsive
	Superficial	Aggressive
	Exploitative	Deceitful
	Unempathic	Lacks the history of conduct disorder in childhood or criminal behavior in adulthood
		ASPD is not as needy of the admiration and envy of others
BPD	Crave attention	NPD has:
		More stable self-image
		Relative lack of self-destructiveness, impulsivity, and abandonment concerns

(continued)

TABLE 12-19   **DSM-IV-TR NARCISSISTIC PERSONALITY DISORDER—Continued**

	Shared Characteristics	Differentiating Characteristics
OCPD	Profess a commitment to perfectionism and believe that others cannot do as well	Self-criticism is present in OCPD while NPD believe that they have achieved perfection
Schizotypal or PPD	Suspiciousness Social withdrawal	These qualities in NPD derive from fears of having imperfections or flaws revealed.

Manic or hypomanic patients may also have associated grandiosity—Traits emerge due to the direct effects of a GMC.
Symptoms that may develop in association with chronic substance use—Only when these traits are inflexible, maladaptive, and persisting and cause significant functional impairment or subjective distress do they constitute NPD.

SOURCE: Adapted from DSM-IV-TR, pp. 714–17.

TABLE 12-20 CULTURE/AGE/GENDER CONSIDERATIONS OF NARCISSISTIC PERSONALITY DISORDER

Culture	Unknown or nonspecific.
Age	May be particulary common in adolescents. Persons with this disorder may have special difficulties adjusting to the onset of physical and occupational limitations that are inherent in the aging process.
Gender	50–75% diagnosed are male.

SOURCE: Adapted from DSM-IV-TR, p. 716.

TABLE 12-21 BIOPSYCHOSOCIAL MANAGEMENT GUIDELINES SPECIFIC TO NARCISSISTIC PERSONALITY DISORDER

Biological	If Axis I disorders, or acute symptoms, psychotropic medications are appropriate.
Psychosocial	In the acute phase, it is best to be prepared for an individual who is entitled and often critical and help-rejecting. This individual thinks he is special and the clinician is not and, therefore, could not possibly understand or help him. He attempts to maintain his self-image as superior. The clinician's role is to be firm, supportive, consistent, and directive. Avoid reinforcing his grandiosity and weakness. The focus should continually be on the problems that led to his crisis and how best to stabilize him. Confrontation is to be avoided. Hospitalization may be necessary if there is severe Axis I overlay and if the patient meets criteria for acute hospitalization. Groups, couples, family therapy: Groups that are specialized to this patient population may be helpful eventually, as a means of practicing and tolerating increased social situations. In groups, the authority of the clinician is less and, therefore, less threatening to the NPD.

Dependent personality disorder (DPD) (Tables 12-25 to 12-27)

Cluster C PDs are anxious and fearful and include:

Obsessive-compulsive personality disorder (OCPD) (Tables 12-28 to 12-30)

Avoidant personality disorder (APD) (Tables 12-22 to 12-24)

TABLE 12-22   DSM-IV-TR AVOIDANT PERSONALITY DISORDER

Prevalence/familial pattern	0.5–1% in general population; 10% in outpatient mental health clinics.
Core	Pattern of social inhibition, feelings of inadequacy, and hypersensitivity to negative evaluation.
Associated symptoms/ comorbidity	• Often vigilantly appraise the movements and expressions of those with whom they come into contact. • Fearful, tense demeanor may elicit derision from others, which confirms their self-doubts. • Anxious that they will react to criticism with blushing or crying. • Described by others as shy, timid, lonely, and isolated. • Major problem is social and occupational functioning. • Low self-esteem and hypersensitivity to refection are associated with restricted interpersonal contacts and social isolation. • Desire affection and acceptance and may fantasize about idealized relationships with others. • Occupationally, may avoid situations that are necessary for job advancement (e.g., public speaking or presentations). • Mood, anxiety disorders, social phobia may co-occur. Other personality disorders such as dependent, BPD, and Cluster A personality disorders may co-occur.
Differential diagnosis	*Social phobia, generalized type*—much overlap here, so much so that they may be alternative conceptualizations of the same or similar conditions. *Panic disorder with agoraphobia*—often co-occurs. However, avoidance in panic disorder typically starts after the onset of panic attacks and may vary based on their frequency and intensity while avoidance in APD tends to have an early onset, an absence of clear precipitants, and a stable course. *Other Personality Disorders:*

PD	Shared Characteristics	Differentiating Characteristics
Dependent personality disorder	Feelings of inadequacy Hypersensitivity to criticism Need for reassurance	Primary focus in DPD is on being taken care of while the primary focus of concern in APD is avoidance of humiliation and rejection.

(continued)

TABLE 12-22   **DSM-IV-TR AVOIDANT PERSONALITY DISORDER—Continued**

PD	Shared Characteristics	Differentiating Characteristics
Schizoid and schizoptypal PDs	Both characterized by social isolation	APD wants to have relationships with others and feel their loneliness deeply while schizoid or schizotypal PDs may prefer social isolation.
PPD	Reluctance to confide in others	In APD this reluctance is due to a fear of being embarrassed or found inadequate rather than to a fear of others' malicious intent.

Personality change due to a GMC—Traits emerge due to the direct effects of a GMC.

Symptoms that may develop in association with chronic substance use—Many may display avoidant personality traits; only when these traits are inflexible, maladaptive, and persisting and cause significant functional impairment or subjective distress do they constitute APD.

SOURCE: Adapted from DSM-IV-TR, pp. 718–21.

TABLE 12-23 CULTURE/AGE/GENDER CONSIDERATIONS OF AVOIDANT PERSONALITY DISORDER

Culture	Variations in the degree to which different cultural and ethnic groups regard diffidence and avoidance as appropriate.
	May be the result of acculturation problems following immigration.
Age	Shyness in children and adolescents may be developmentally appropriate; do not be too quick to diagnose.
Gender	Equally frequent in males and females.

SOURCE: Adapted from DSM-IV-TR, p. 719.

TABLE 12-24 BIOPSYCHOSOCIAL MANAGEMENT GUIDELINES SPECIFIC TO AVOIDANT PERSONALITY DISORDER

Biological	Acute symptoms.
	Axis I disorders such as comorbid disorders listed in Table 12-20.
Psychosocial	Acute presentations may be precipitated by stressful situations, which overwhelm the patient's coping repertoire.
	Focus on problem solving. Know that these patients devalue themselves and may not bother to give complete answers to questions; they may be vague and leave out information.
	Individual psychotherapy.
	Group particularly geared for this population as a way of exposing and increasing tolerance to discomfort in social situations.
	Family, couples.
	Self-help; such patients are highly uncomfortable and anxious in groups so this is probably ineffective simply due to their likely avoidance of such groups.

TABLE 12-25   **DSM-IV-TR DEPENDENT PERSONALITY DISORDER**

Prevalence/familial pattern	Among the most frequently reported in mental health clinics.
Core	Pattern of submissive and clinging behavior related to an excessive need to be taken care of.
Associated symptoms/ comorbidity	Often characterized by pessimism and self-doubt. Belittle their abilities and assets. May constantly refer to themselves as "stupid." Criticism and disapproval are seen as proof of their worthlessness and they lose faith in themselves. Seek overprotection and dominance from others. Occupational functioning may be impaired if self-initiation is required, and they may avoid positions of responsibility and become anxious when faced with decisions. Social relations are limited. Mood disorders, anxiety disorders, and adjustment disorders may co-occur. Other personality disorders especially BPD, avoidant and histrionic PDs, may co-occur. Chronic physical illness or separation anxiety disorder in childhood or adolescence may predispose the individual to the development of this disorder.
Differential diagnosis	*Axis I disorders such as mood disorders, panic disorder, and agoraphobia* may create dependency. *GMCs* may also create dependency. DPD has an early-onset, chronic course and a pattern of behavior that does not occur exclusively during an Axis I or Axis III disorder. *Other Personality Disorders:*

PD	Shared Characteristics	Differentiating Characteristics
BPD	Fear of abandonment with feelings of emotional emptiness, rage, and demand	DPD reacts with increasing appeasement and submissiveness and urgently seeks a replacement relationship. BPD has a typical patten of unstable and intense relationships.
HPD	Strong need for reassurance and approval May appear child-like and clinging	DPD is more self-effacing and docile while HPD is gregarious, flamboyant, with active demands for attention.

(continued)

TABLE 12-25   **DSM-IV-TR DEPENDENT PERSONALITY DISORDER—Continued**

PD	Shared Characteristics	Differentiating Characteristics
APD	Feelings of inadequacy Hypersensitivity to criticism Need for reassurance	APD have a strong fear of humiliation and rejection while DPD have a pattern of seeking and maintaining connections to important others rather than avoiding and withdrawing from relationships
	Personality change due to a GMC—Traits emerge due to the direct effects of a GMC. *Symptoms that may develop in association with chronic substance use*—Traits emerge due to the direct effects of substance use. *Display of dependent personality traits*—Only when these traits are inflexible, maladaptive, persistent, and cause significant distress and/or impairment should the individual be diagnosed with DPD.	

SOURCE: Adapted from DSM-IV-TR, pp. 721–25.

TABLE 12-26 CULTURE/AGE/GENDER CONSIDERATIONS OF DEPENDENT PERSONALITY DISORDER

Culture	The degree to which dependent behaviors are considered to be appropriate varies substantially across different age and sociocultural groups. Must consider cultural factors in evaluating the diagnostic threshold of each criterion (e.g., an emphasis on passivity, politeness, and deferential treatment is characteristic of some cultures).
Age	Consider the developmental stage and whether it is appropriate.
Gender	Diagnosed more frequently in females but may be similar prevalence rates for male and female.

Source: Adapted from DSM-IV-TR, p. 723.

TABLE 12-27 BIOPSYCHOSOCIAL MANAGEMENT GUIDELINES SPECIFIC TO DEPENDENT PERSONALITY DISORDER

Biological	Treat acute symptoms and identifiable Axis I disorders. Careful monitoring of medications due to vulnerability to sedative drug abuse and overdose. Resist temptation to overprescribe.
Psychosocial	In the acute phase, ego-bolstering, supportive techniques that are solution-focused are preferred.
	Simple matter-of-fact approach. Such patients are needy, make repeated requests for attention, and may seem compliant but are more typically passively help-rejecting. Still it is important to *not* dismiss physical complaints.
	Clear boundaries, clear limits delineated from the outset and followed.
	This disorder differs from the other PDs in that long-term psychotherapy is contraindicated because it would only reinforce dependency traits. Instead short-term, solution-focused supportive therapy is encouraged, with clinician avoiding rescuer role and being aware that such patients often elicit irritation due to their clinging, needy behaviors.
	Family/couples group.
	Self-help—if specific to this disorder and in addition to other treatment modalities—may be helpful.

TABLE 12-28 **DSM-IV-TR OBSESSIVE-COMPULSIVE PERSONALITY DISORDER**

Prevalence/familial pattern	1% in community samples 2–10% in mental health clinic samples
Core	Pattern of preoccupation with orderliness, perfectionism, and control.
Associated symptoms/ comorbidity	Difficulty deciding how to prioritize tasks and/or the best way to approach a task—thus they may never get started on or complete anything. Prone to become upset or angry in situations they cannot control physically or interpersonally but rarely express anger directly or it is expressed out of proportion to the triggering situation. Display deference to authorities they respect and excessive resistance to authorities they do not respect. Express affection in a highly controlled or stilted fashion. Uncomfortable with others who are emotionally expressive. Everyday relationships have a formal or serious quality. Stiff, hold themselves back until they are sure that whatever they say will be perfect. Occupational difficulties arise in new situations that demand flexibility and compromise. Co-occurring anxiety disorders (e.g., GAD, OCD, social and specific phobias). Though majority of patients with OCD do not have OCPD, OCPD traits often overlap with type A personality characteristics (preoccupation with work, competitiveness, and time urgency). Also may be an association between OCPD and mood and eating disorders.
Differential diagnosis	*OCD*: easily distinguished from OCPD by the presence of obsessions and/or compulsions but an individual may meet the criteria for both. *Other Personality Disorders:*

PD	Shared Characteristics	Differentiating Characteristics
NPD	Perfectionism Belief that others cannot do things as well	NPD believe they have achieved perfection while OCPD are usually self-critical.
ASPD	Lack generosity	ASPD indulge themselves while OCPD adopt a miserly spending style toward themselves and others.
Schizoid PD	Formality Social detachment	OCPD stems from discomfort with emotions and excessive devotion to work.

(continued)

PD	Shared Characteristics	Differentiating Characteristics
		In SPD, this stems from a fundamental lack of capacity for intimacy.
		Personality change due to a GMC—Traits emerge due to the direct effects of a GMC. *Symptoms that may develop in association with chronic substance use*—Traits emerge due to the direct effects of substance use. *Obsessive-compulsive personality traits in moderation*—may be especially adaptive in situations that reward high performance. Only if such traits are inflexible, maladaptive, and persisting and cause significant impairment or subjective distress do they constitute OCPD.

Source: Adapted from DSM-IV-TR, pp. 725–29.

TABLE 12-29 CULTURE/AGE/GENDER CONSIDERATIONS OF OBSESSIVE-COMPULSIVE PERSONALITY DISORDER

Culture	Consider culture; do not include those behaviors that reflect habits, customs, or interpersonal styles culturally sanctioned by the individual's reference group; certain cultures place substantial emphasis on work and productivity.
Age	Nonspecific.
Gender	Diagnosed twice as often among males.

SOURCE: Adapted from DSM-IV-TR, p. 728.

TABLE 12-30 BIOPSYCHOSOCIAL MANAGEMENT GUIDELINES SPECIFIC TO OBSESSIVE-COMPULSIVE PERSONALITY DISORDER

Biological	Treat acute symptoms and identifiable Axis I disorders.
Psychosocial	• Such patients may present in an acute phase due to situational stressors—job change, marital and family strife—that have overwhelmed their coping mechanisms.
	• Bolster their existing coping strategies while teaching new ones. But be aware that these are patients who tend to quickly reject treatment options that do not fit within their comfort zone.
	• These patients are black-and-white thinkers; citing a study or recent literature in support of your proposed treatment may help the process, but even then, do not personalize rejection. Stick to facts.
	• Expect attacks on your professionalism and knowledge and do not engage in struggles that focus away from the patient or engage in long intellectual discussions that collude with the patient's desire to distance from feelings.
	In groups, such patients are typically ostracized for pointing out others' deficits.
	Individual therapy should focus on current social and coping skills. Reinforce these and teach new ones. Reinforce healthy feeling states, help with identifying feelings.

DISSOCIATIVE IDENTITY DISORDER (TABLES 12-31 TO 12-33)

TABLE 12-31   DSM-IV-TR DISSOCIATIVE IDENTITY DISORDER (FORMERLY MULTIPLE PD)

Prevalence/familial pattern	*Controversial. Some clinicians believe that the increase in reported cases in the United States in recent years is due to increased awareness; others believe that the syndrome is overdiagnosed in highly suggestible individuals by highly gullible clinicians.* May be more common in first-degree biological relatives of persons with the disorder than in the general population.
Core symptoms	Presence of two or more distinct identities or personality states (each with its own relatively enduring pattern of perceiving, relating to, and thinking about the environment and self).
Associated symptoms/ comorbidity	Severe physical and sexual abuse in childhood. Repetitive relationships involving physical and/or sexual abuse. Mood, substance-related, sexual, eating, or sleep disorders. Other Axis I disorders such as mood, anxiety (PTSD), psychotic disorders. Comorbid personality disorders such as BPD. Such patients score toward the upper end of the distribution on measures of hypnotizability and dissociative capacity. Reports of variations in physiological function across identity states, e.g., differences in visual acuity, pain tolerance, symptoms of asthma, sensitivity to allergens, response of blood glucose to insulin.

Differential diagnosis	*Personality disorder due to a GMC*—Traits emerge due to the direct effects of a GMC (e.g., complex partial seizures).
	Personality disorder due to chronic substance use—Traits emerge due to the direct effects of a substance.
	Other PDs
	Axis I disorders such as psychotic disorders
	Malingering
	Other dissociative disorders such as:
	    Dissociative amnesia
	    Dissociative fugue
	    Depersonaization disorder
	    Dissociative disorder NOS
	    Factitious disorder

SOURCE: Adapted from DSM-IV-TR, pp. 526–29.

TABLE 12-32 **CULTURE/AGE/GENDER FEATURES OF DISSOCIATIVE IDENTITY DISORDER**

Culture	Consider cultural variables; this has been found in individuals from various cultures around the world.
Age	Limited data in childhood.
Gender	Females > males.

SOURCE: Adapted from DSM-IV-TR, p. 528.

TABLE 12-33 **BIOPSYCHOSOCIAL MANAGEMENT GUIDELINES SPECIFIC TO DISSOCIATIVE IDENTITY DISORDER**

Biological	• Acute symptoms reduction. • Specific Axis I disorder. • Long-term medication is usually not recommended because these patients have particular problems with impulse control, and there is risk for overdose. • If used, should be carefully monitored.
Psychosocial	In the acute phase, support, ego bolstering, solution-focused. Main goal of longer-term therapy is the integration of the various alters into one cohesive personality.

DSM-IV-TR PERSONALITY DISORDER NOT OTHERWISE SPECIFIED

The individual's personality pattern meets the general criteria of personality disorder and traits of several personality disorders are present but criteria for a specific PD are not met. The individual's personality pattern meets the general criteria for a personality disorder, but the individual is not considered to have a personality disorder that is not included in the classification (e.g., passive-aggressive personality disorder).

COLLABORATIVE LONGITUDINAL PERSONALITY DISORDERS STUDY

Bender et al. started with a hypothesis: Patients with personality disorders utilize more and a broader range of mental health services than those without personality disorders.

They selected 698 treatment-seeking patients aged 18–45 at several treatment sites. These patients were interviewed as well as given personality testing and all were divided into five cells: avoidant, schizoptypal, borderline, OCPD, and MDD without PD.

Based on extensive interviews with the patients, the hypothesis was confirmed, with BPD patients utilizing virtually every known treatment including the most restrictive hospitalization, day treatment, outpatient individual, couples, family, and group therapies. Of patients with a diagnosis of schizotypal who were seeking treatment, 29% also met criteria for BPD and these patients had a high utilization pattern. Avoidant patients had a low utilization of mental health services. OCPD patients had a higher use of individual therapy. Patients with MDD without PD had less use.

Of interest was that 65% of patients met criteria for two or more Axis II disorders; of patients with Axis II disorders, comorbidity with an Axis I disorder was 98%.

BIBLIOGRAPHY

American Psychiatric Association. *Practice Guidelines for the Treatment of Patients with Borderline Personality Disorder.* http://www.psych.org.

Bender D, et al. Treatment Utilization by Patients with Personality Disorders. *American Journal of Psychiatry* 158 (February 2001): 295–302.

Diagnostic and Statistical Manual of Mental Disorders, 4th ed., Text Revision (DSM-IV-TR). Washington, DC: American Psychiatric Association, 2000.

Othmer E, Othmer SC. *The Clinical Interview Using DSM-IV-TR, Vol. 2: The Difficult Patient.* Washington, DC: American Psychiatric Publishing, 2001.

Weston D. Divergences between Clinical and Research Methods for Accessing Personality Disorders: Implications for Research and the Evolution of Axis II. *American Journal of Psychiatry* 154 (1997): 895–903.

Westen D, Arkowitz-Western L. Limitations of Axis II in Diagnosing Personality Pathology in Clinical Practice. *American Journal of Psychiatry* 155 (1998): 1767–71.

Zimmerman M, Mattia JI. Differences between Clinical and Research Practices in Diagnosing Borderline Personality Disorder. *American Journal of Psychiatry* 156 (1999): 1570–74.

INDEX

Anxiolytic-related disorders, 167, 168–169*t*
  culture, age, and gender features of, 169*t*
  DSM-IV-TR diagnostic criteria, 170*t*
Avoidant personality disorder
  biopsychosocial management guidelines
    specific to, 217*t*
  culture/age/gender considerations of,
    217*t*
  DSM-IV-TR criteria for, 215–216*t*

B

Barbiturates, 167
Behavioral emergencies
  defined, 24
  medications in, 25–28
Benzene, 156
Benzodiazepines, 167
Benzoylecgonine, 151*t*
Beta-blockers, 144*t*
Biological treatment, 23–40
  for alcohol disorders, 143–144*t*
  for amphetamine disorders, 146*t*
  for antisocial personality disorders,
    204*t*
  for avoidant personality disorder, 217*t*
  for borderline personality disorder, 208*t*
  chemical restraint versus, 24
  for cocaine use disorders, 152*t*
  for dependent personality disorder, 220*t*
  for dissociative identity disorder, 225*t*
  for histrionic personality disorder, 211*t*
  medications
    antianxiety, 35, 35*t*, 36*t*, 37*t*
    anticholinergic, 34, 34*t*
    antidepressant, 38, 38*t*
    antipsychotic, 30, 31*t*, 32*t*, 33*t*
    in behavioral emergencies, 25–28
    mood stabilizing, 39*t*
  for narcissistic personality disorder, 214*t*
  for obsessive-compulsive personality
    disorder, 223*t*
  for opioid-induced disorders, 163–164*t*
  risk management strategies in, 40
  for schizophrenia and other psychotic
    disorders, 187–188*t*
  for schizotypal personality disorder, 201*t*
  strategies if inadequate response to initial
    interventions, 29, 29*t*

Biopsychosocial management guidelines
  for antisocial personality disorder, 204*t*
  for anxiety disorders, 123*t*
  for avoidant personality disorder, 217*t*
  for borderline personality disorder, 208–209*t*
  for dependent personality disorder, 220*t*
  for dissociative identity disorder, 225*t*
  for histrionic personality disorder, 211*t*
  for mood disorders, 107*t*
  for narcissistic personality disorder, 214*t*
  for obsessive-compulsive personality
    disorder, 223*t*
  for schizotypal personality disorder, 201*t*
Biopsychosocial model, 41
Bipolar disorders, 92, 103–107
  biopsychosocial treatment of, 107*t*
  bipolar I, 103–104*t*
  bipolar II, 105*t*
  in children, 103
  cultural considerations in, 103
  cyclothymic disorders, 106*t*
  in elderly, 103
  not otherwise specified, 107*t*
  specifiers, 103*t*
  suicide and, 91
  in women, 103
Blood alcohol levels, 19–20
  in nontolerant alcohol-intoxicated patient,
    140*t*
Borderline personality disorder
  biopsychosocial management guidelines
    specific to, 208–209*t*
  culture/age/gender considerations of, 207*t*
  DSM-IV-TR criteria for, 205–206*t*
Breach of duty, 50
Breathalyzer levels, 19–20
Brief psychotic disorder, DSM-IV-TR criteria
  for, 181–182*t*
Bulimia nervosa, 113*t*
Buspirone, 144*t*

C

Caffeine-related disorders, 147, 147*t*
  culture, age, and gender features of, 147*t*
Cannabis-related disorders, 148, 148*t*
Carbamates, 167
Cardiovascular syndrome, 9*t*
Casuistry, 60

Environment, assuring safe, for emergency evaluation, 16
Epidemiologic Catchment Area (ECA) studies, 127
Ethical dilemma, 60
Ethical reasoning, 60
Ethical workup, 62, 62*t*
Ethics, 60. *See also* Psychiatric ethics of care, 60

F

Family therapies, 136
Financial factors, ethics and, 63
Flashbacks, 154*t*
Folie à deux, DSM-IV-TR criteria for, 182*t*
Freebasing, 149

G

Gastric emptying, 10
Gastric lavage, 10
Gender considerations
    for alcohol-related disorders, 142*t*
    for amphetamine-related disorders, 145*t*
    for antisocial personality disorder, 204*t*
    for anxiolytic-related disorders, 169*t*
    for avoidant personality disorder, 217*t*
    for borderline personality disorder, 207*t*
    for caffeine-related disorders, 147*t*
    for cocaine-related disorders, 152*t*
    for delusional disorder, 180*t*
    for dependent personality disorder, 220*t*
    for dissociative identity disorder, 225*t*
    for hallucinogen-related disorders, 155*t*
    for histrionic personality disorder, 211*t*
    for hypnotic-related disorders, 169*t*
    for inhalant-related disorders, 158*t*
    for narcissistic personality disorder, 214*t*
    for obsessive-compulsive personality disorder, 223*t*
    for opioid-related disorders, 162*t*
    for paranoid personality disorder, 195*t*
    for phencyclidine-related disorders, 166*t*
    for potentially suicidal patients, 73
    for schizoaffective disorder, 178*t*
    for schizoid personality disorder, 198*t*

for schizotypal personality disorder, 201*t*
    for sedative-related disorders, 169*t*
Generalized anxiety disorder (GAD), 120*t*
    anxiety disorder due to, 121*t*
General medical conditions, 79*t*
    agitation due to, 28*f*
    DSM-IV-TR criteria for psychotic disorder due to, 183–184*t*
    features suggestive of, 5*t*
    mood disorder due to, 100*t*
    risk of violence with, 78*t*
General organic mental syndromes, 6*t*
Global Assessment of Functioning (GAF), 48
Group therapies, 136

H

Hallucinations
    command, 79*t*
    persistent auditory, 186
Hallucinogen persisting perception disorder, 154*t*
Hallucinogen-related disorders, 153–155, 155*t*
    culture, age, and gender features of, 155*t*
Health care rationing, ethics and, 63
Heroin, 159
History
    current social, 16
    from other sources, 20
    past medical, 7–8, 17
    of present illness, 7, 16
    psychiatric, for emergency evaluation, 17*t*
    weapons, 85*t*
Histrionic personality disorder, 191
    biopsychosocial management guidelines specific to, 211*t*
    culture/age/gender considerations of, 211*t*
    DSM-IV-TR criteria for, 210*t*
Homeless shelters, referrals to, 20–21
Homicidal threats, suicide risk in persons making, 88
Hospitalization, 137*t*
    decision for, 20
    involuntary, 55–57, 56*t*
        decision process for, 20
    partial, 137*t*

S

Schizoaffective disorder
  culture/age/gender features of, 178*t*
  DSM-IV-TR criteria for, 178*t*
Schizoid personality disorder
  culture/age/gender considerations of, 198*t*
  DSM-IV-TR criteria for, 196–197*t*
Schizophrenia, 113*t*, 172
  culture/age/gender considerations of, 177*t*
  definitions, 172
  DSM-IV-TR criteria for, 173–176*t*
  emergency assessment and management of, 186, 187–188*t*
  negative symptoms, 172
  positive symptoms, 172
  risk of violence with, 77*t*
Schizotypal personality disorder
  biopsychosocial management guidelines specific to, 201*t*
  culture/age/gender considerations of, 201*t*
  DSM-IV-TR criteria for, 199–200*t*
Seclusion, 54
  contraindications to, 54*t*
  controversy over, 55
  indications for, 54*t*
Security, working with, and potentially violent patients, 80
Sedative hypnotic agents, 9*t*
Sedative-related disorders, 167, 168–169*t*
  culture, age, and gender features of, 169*t*
  DSM-IV-TR diagnostic criteria, 170*t*
Self-help groups, 136
Serial sevens, 18
Serial threes, 18
Shared psychotic disorder, DSM-IV-TR criteria for, 182*t*
Social Anxiety Disorder (SAD), 113–114*t*
Social phobia, 113*t*, 114*t*
  biopsychosocial treatment of, 123*t*
Socioeconomically deprived patients, suicide risk in, 72
Stimulants, 145
STP, 153
Substance-induced anxiety disorder, 122*t*
Substance-induced mood disorder, 92, 101–102*t*
Substance-induced psychotic disorder, DSM-IV-TR criteria for, 185*t*

Substance intoxication, agitation due to, 27*f*
Substance use disorders, 127–170
  alcohol-related, 138–144, 141*t*
    alcohol-induced persisting amnesic disorder (Korsakoff's syndrome), 140*t*
    blood alcohol concentrations correlated with typical presentation in nontolerant alcohol-intoxicated patient, 140*t*
    culture, age, and gender features of, 142*t*
    dementia, 140*t*
    DSM-IV-TR diagnostic criteria, 139*t*
    emergency assessment and management, 143–144*t*
    hallucinosis, 140*t*
    intoxication, 139*t*
    intoxication delirium, 140*t*
    not otherwise specified, 140*t*
    Wernicke's encephalopathy, 140*t*
    withdrawal, 139*t*
    withdrawal delirium, 140*t*
    withdrawal seizures, 140*t*
  amphetamine-related disorders, 145–146, 145*t*
    culture, age, and gender features of, 145*t*
    emergency assessment and management, 146*t*
  appropriate choice of treatment settings, 137*t*
  associated features of dependence, abuse, intoxication, and withdrawal, 130–135*t*
  caffeine-related disorders, 147, 147*t*
    culture, age, and gender features of, 147*t*
  cannabis-related disorders, 148, 148*t*
  classification of, 127–128
  cocaine-related disorders, 149, 151*t*
    culture, age, and gender features of, 152*t*
    emergency assessment and management of, 152*t*
    intoxication, 150*t*
    withdrawal, 150*t*
  DSM-IV-TR criteria for, 128
    for substance abuse, 129*t*
    for substance dependence, 128*t*
    for substance intoxication, 129*t*
    for substance withdrawal, 129*t*
  general management/approach in emergency phase, 136–137
  hallucinogen-related disorders, 153–155, 155*t*
    culture, age, and gender features of, 155*t*
    DSM-IV-TR diagnostic criteria, 154*t*

INDEX   **237**